This book belongs to:

....

Please leave a review because we would love to hear your feedback, opinions and advice to create better products and services for you!

You are greatly appreciated!

HUMAN ANATOMY

- RESPIRATORY
- CIRCULATORY
- DIGESTIVE
- URINARY
- NERVOUS
- SKELETON

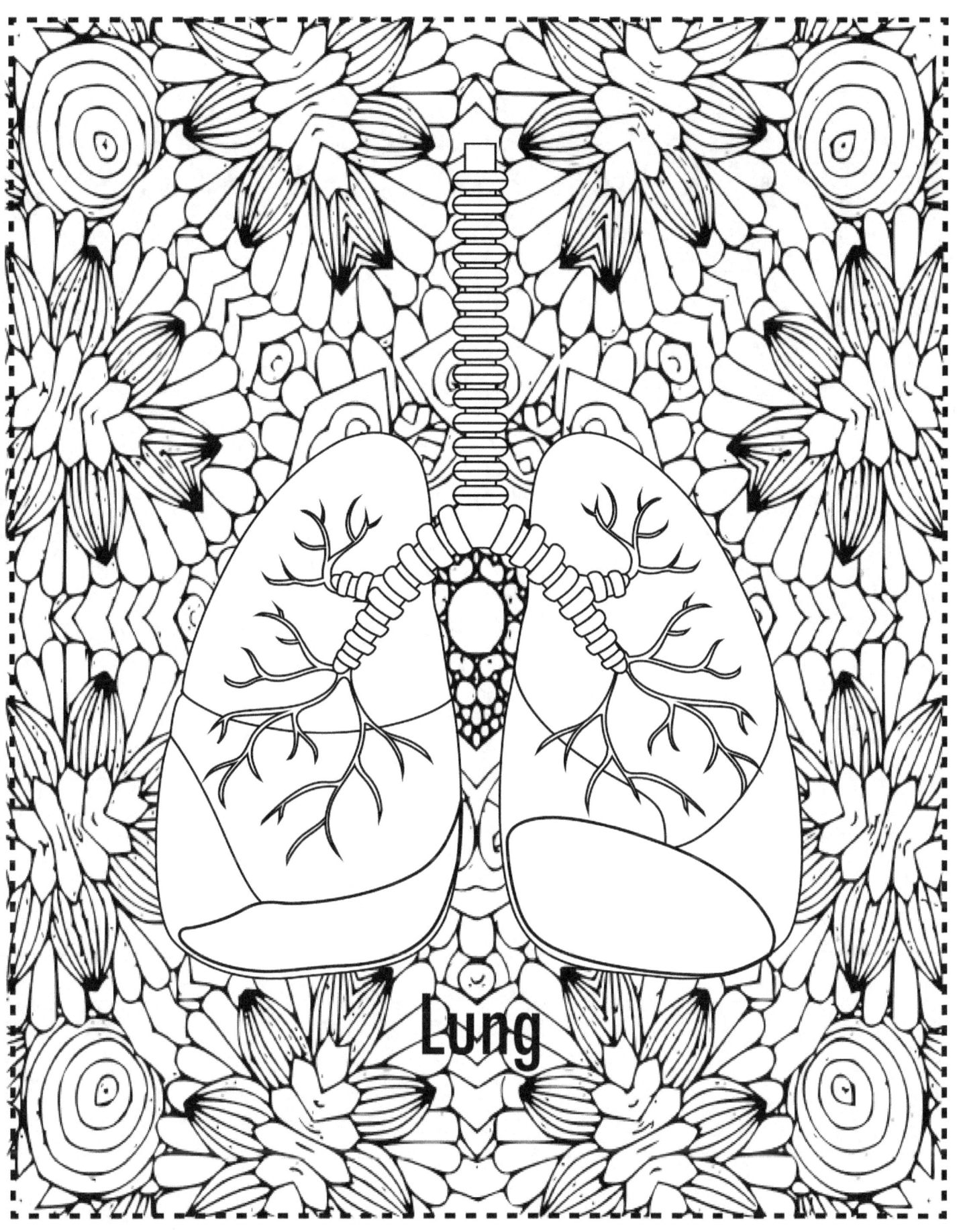

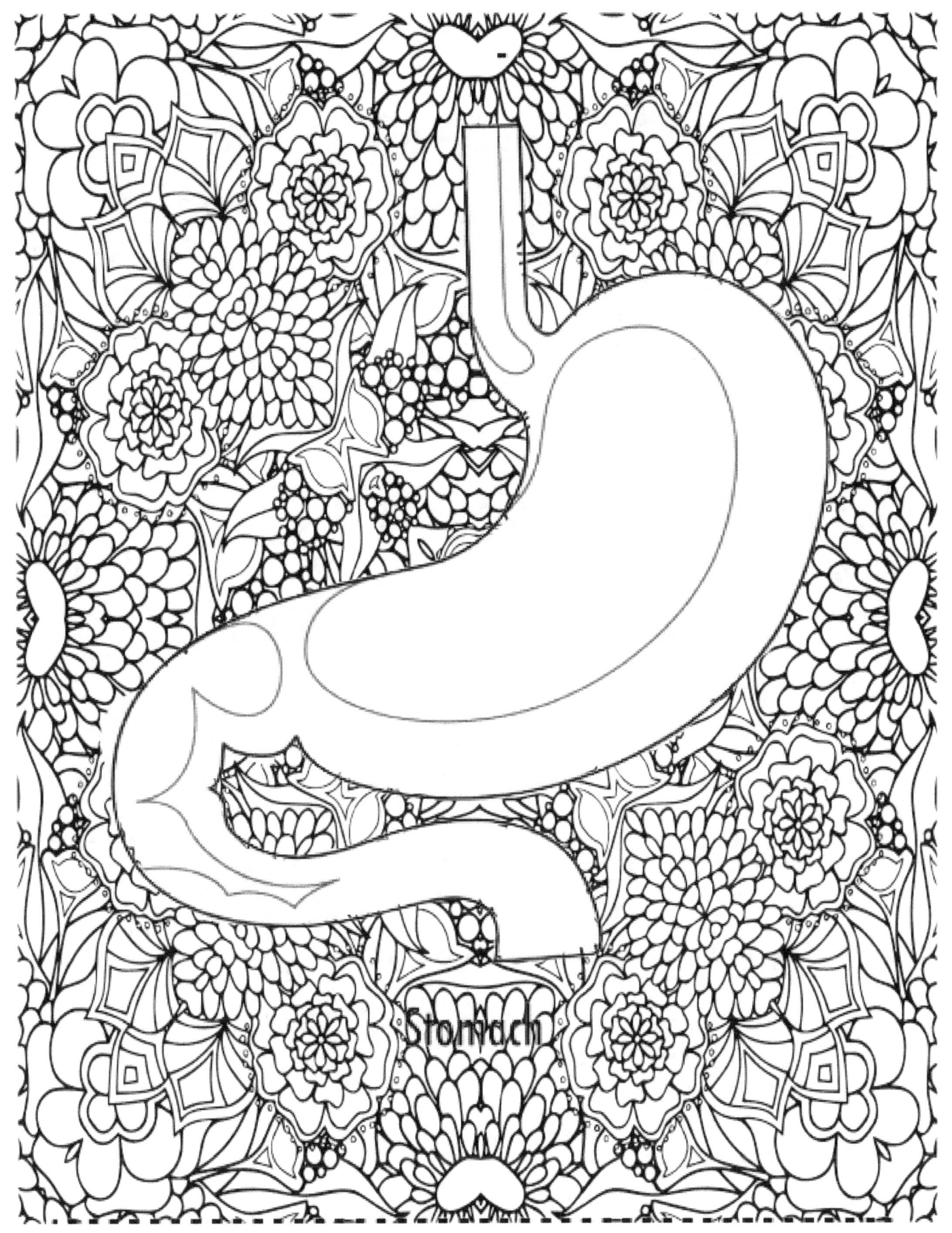

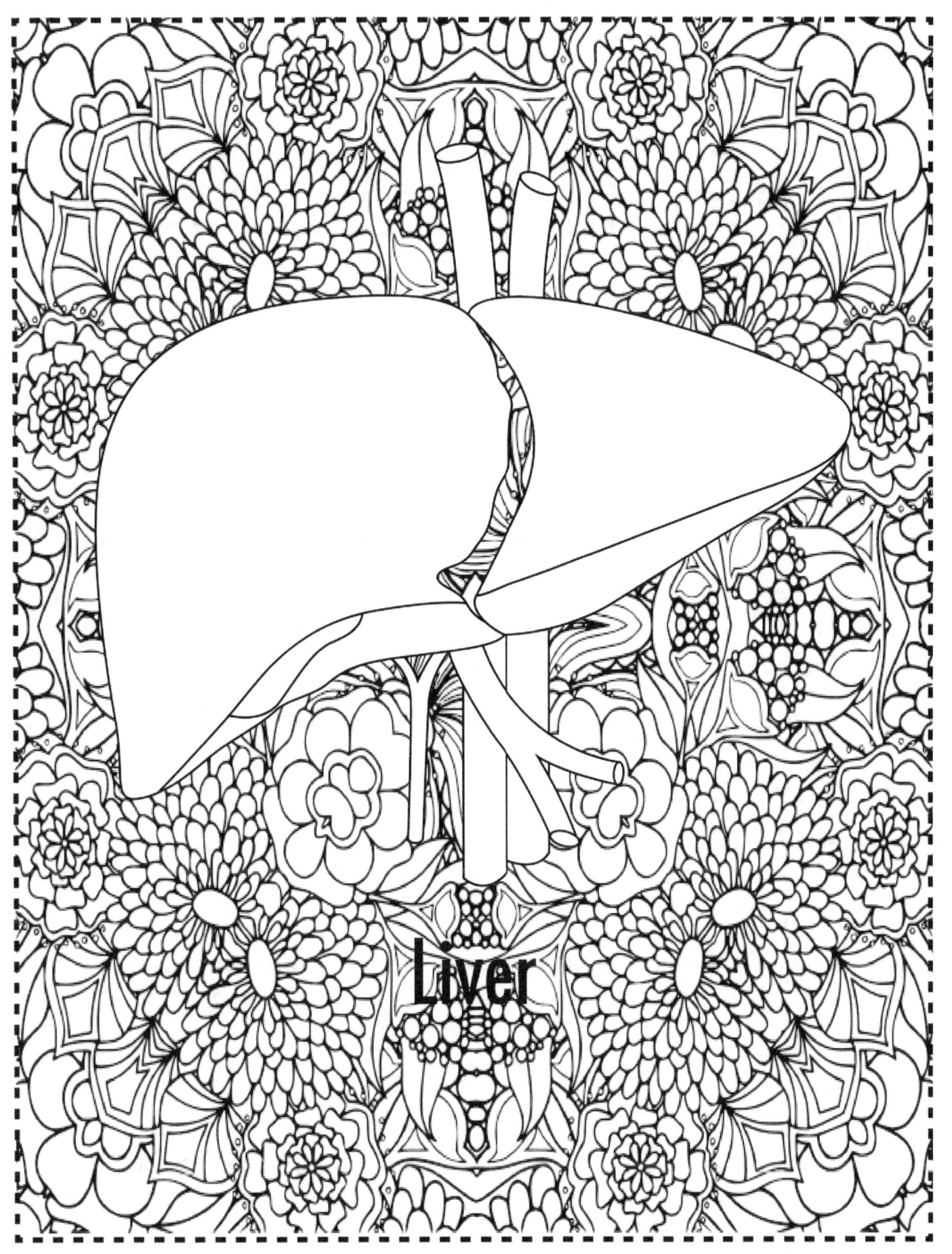

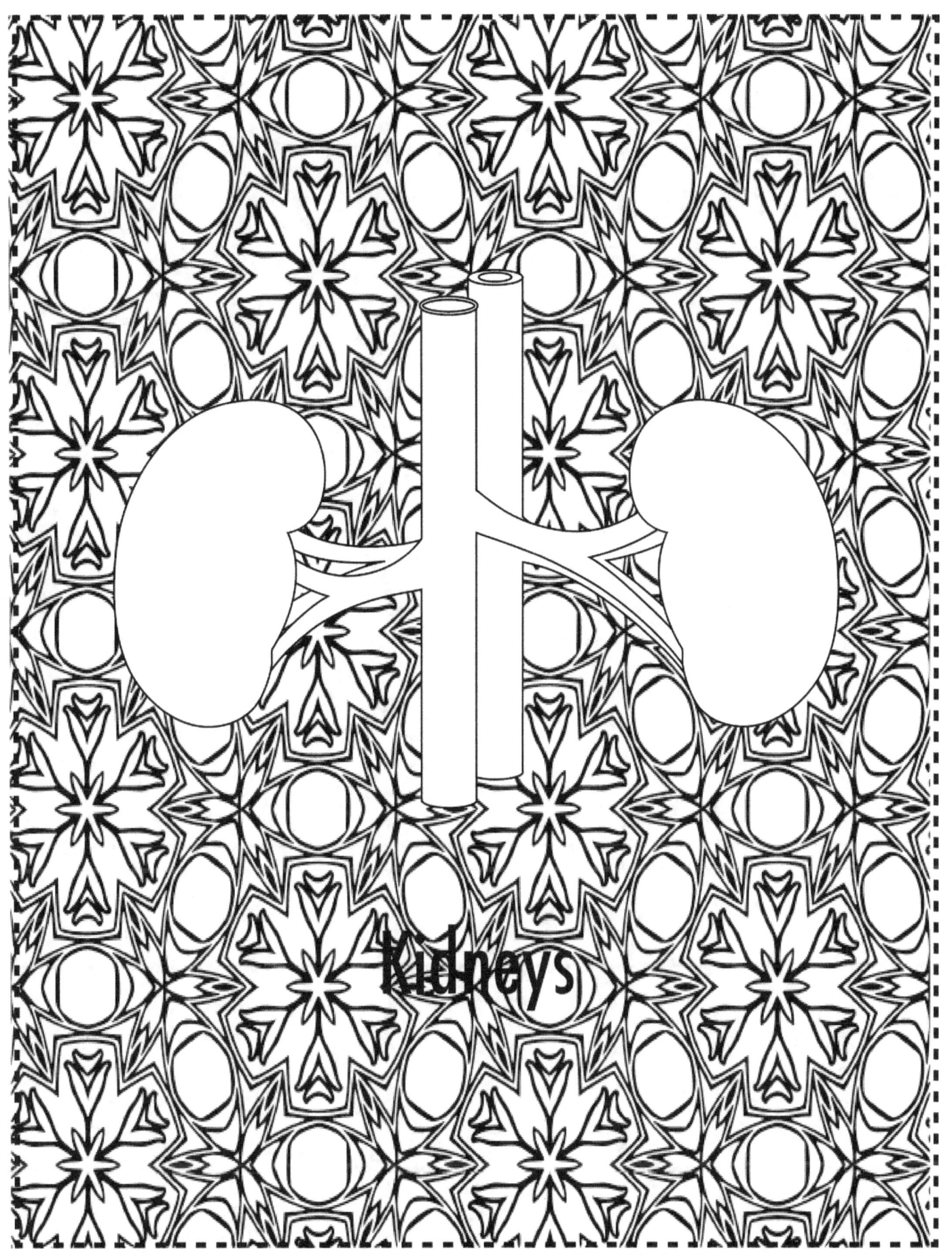

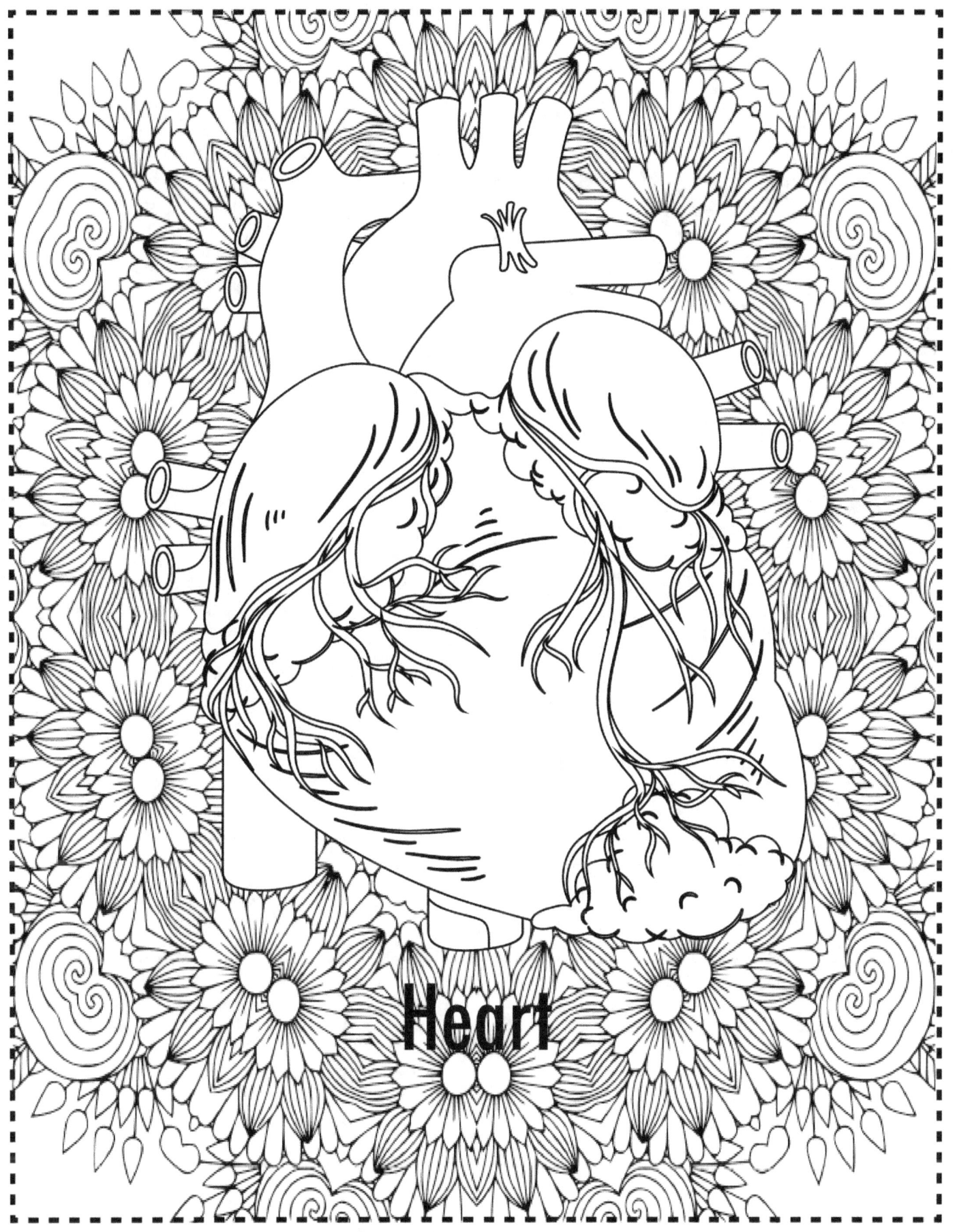

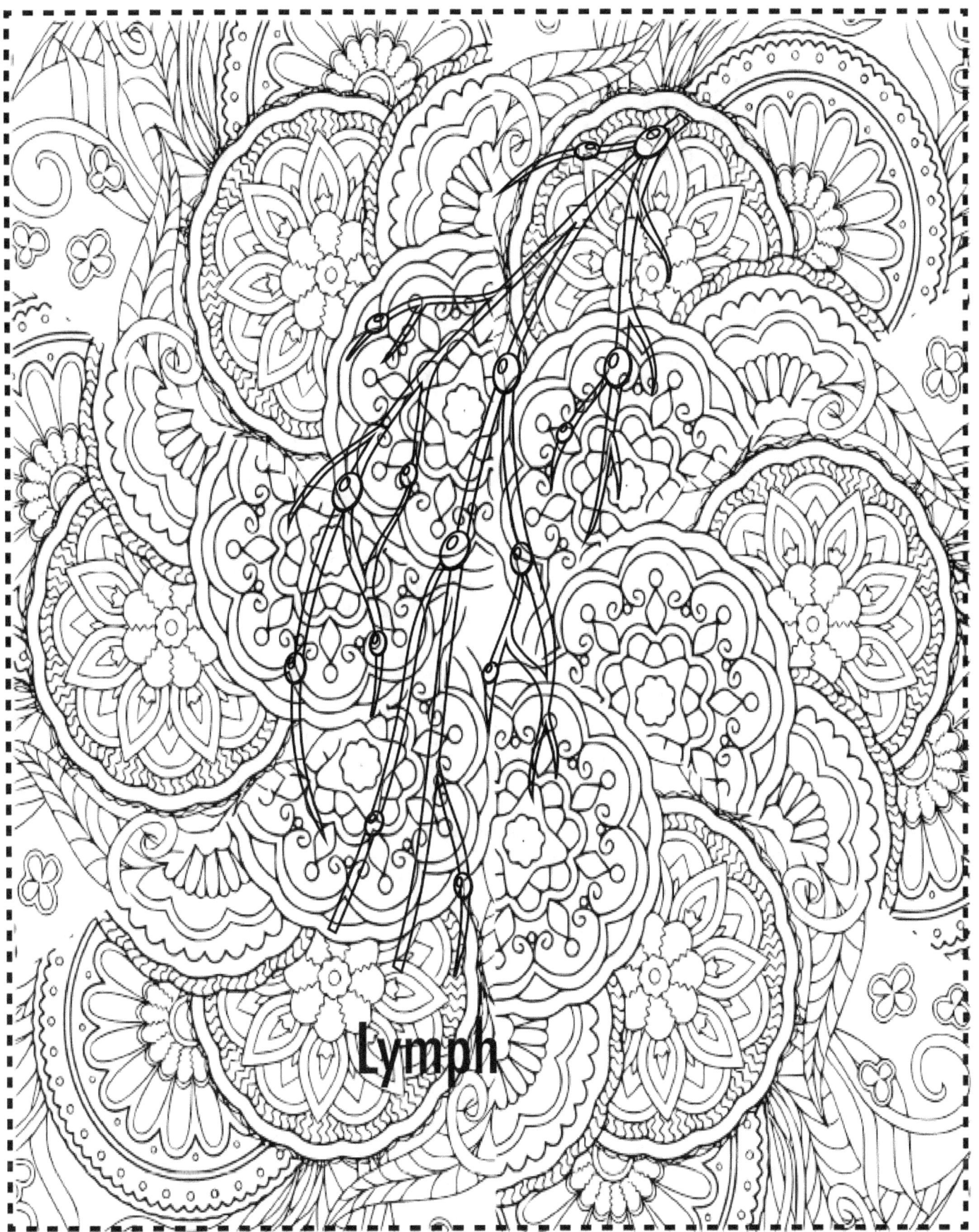

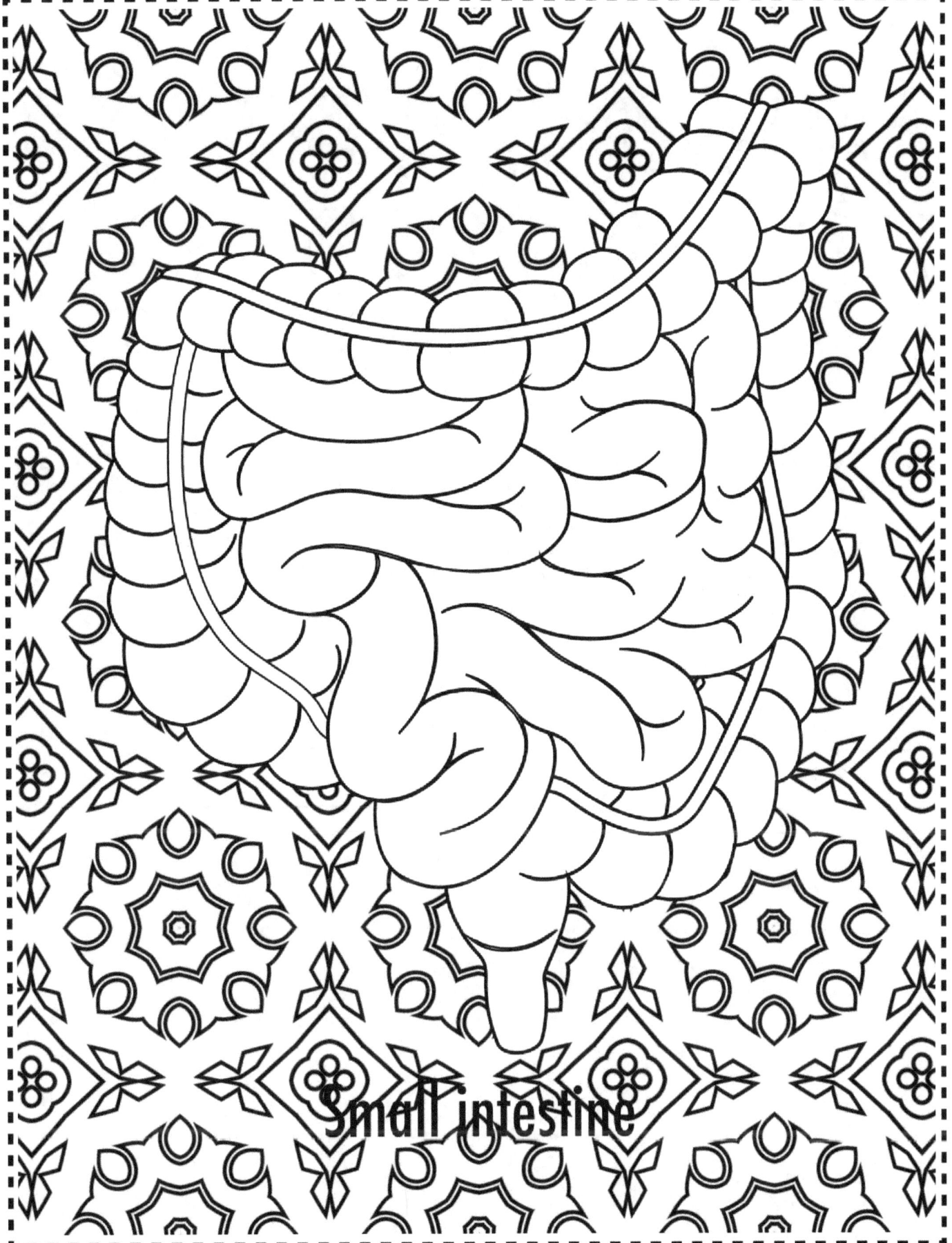

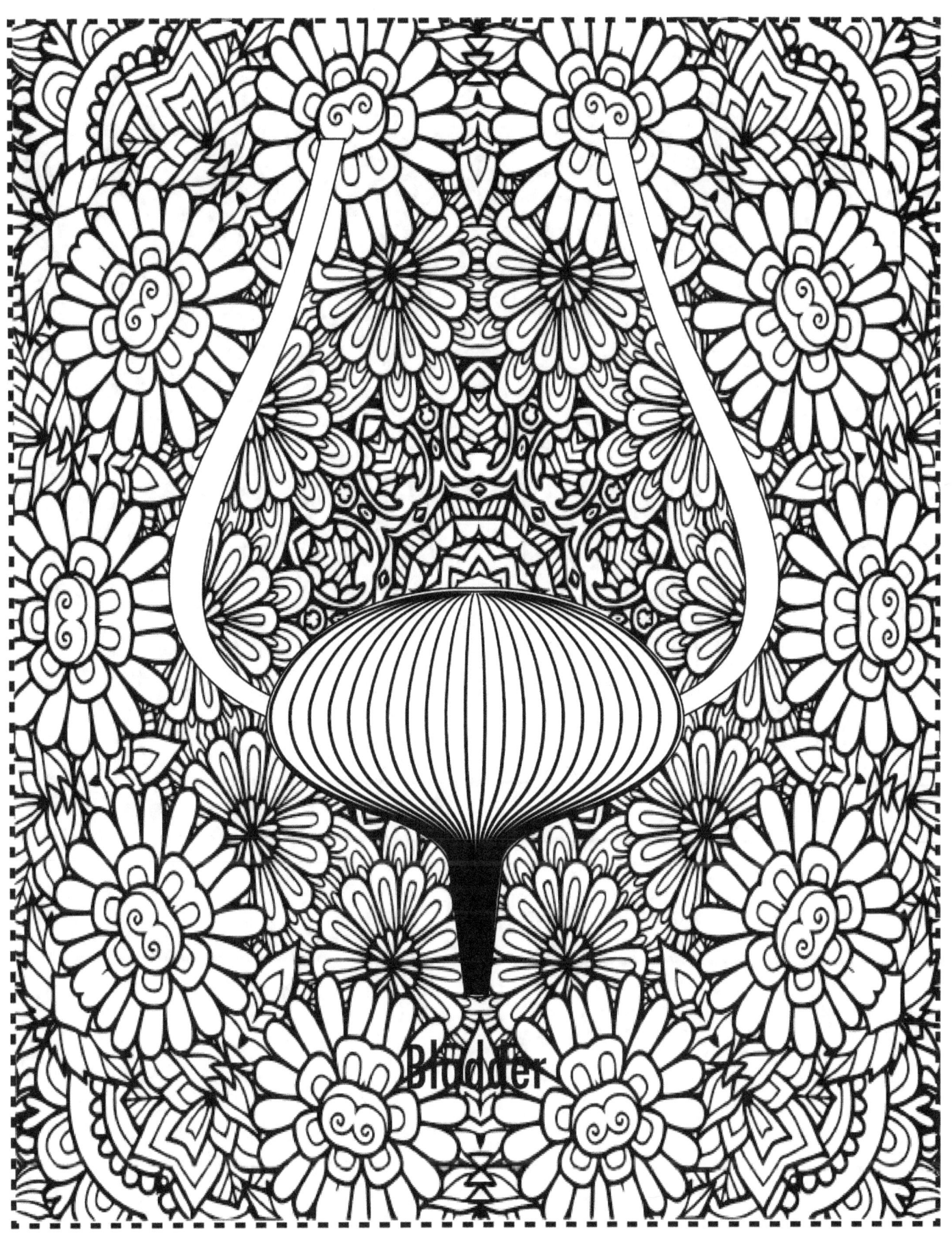

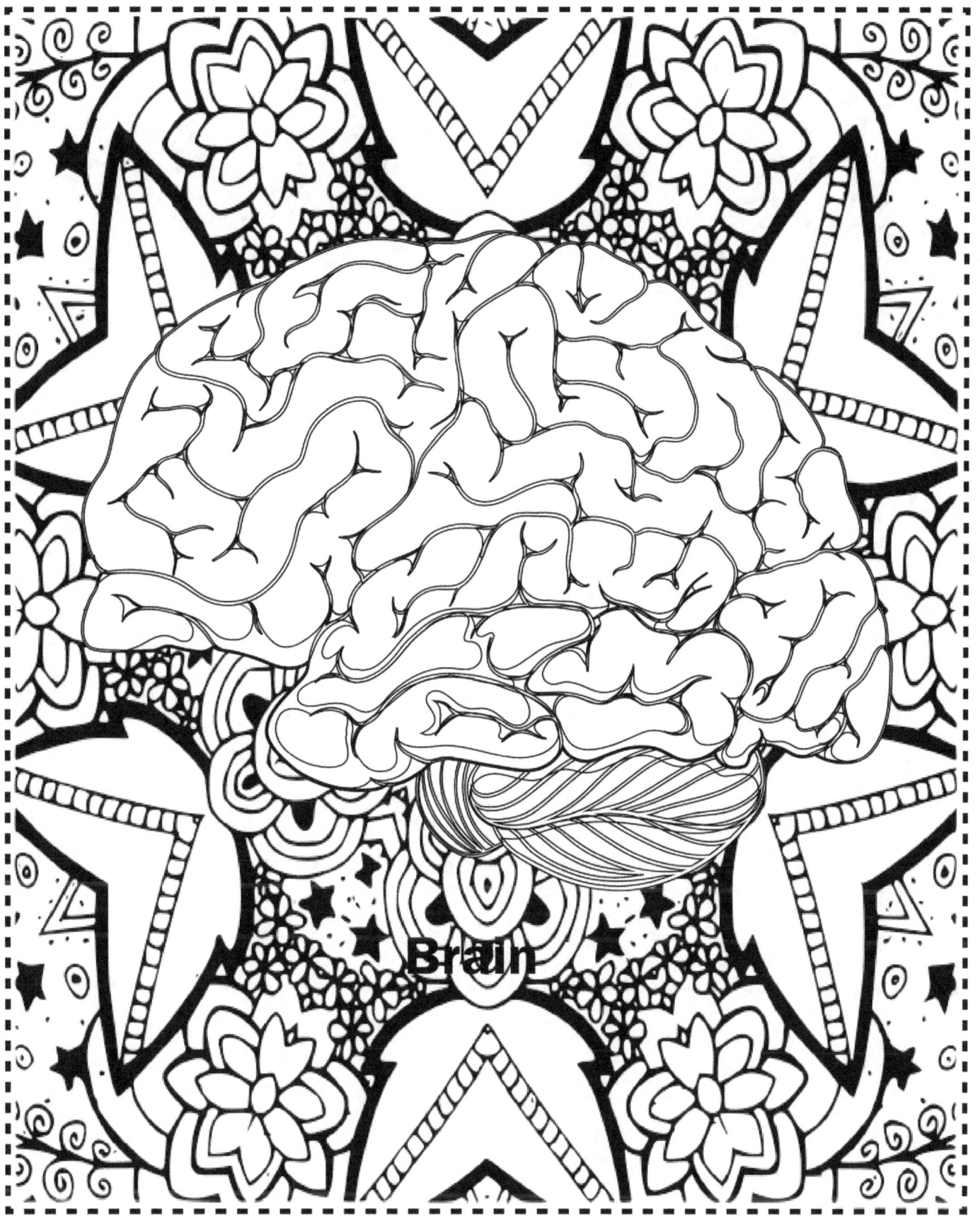

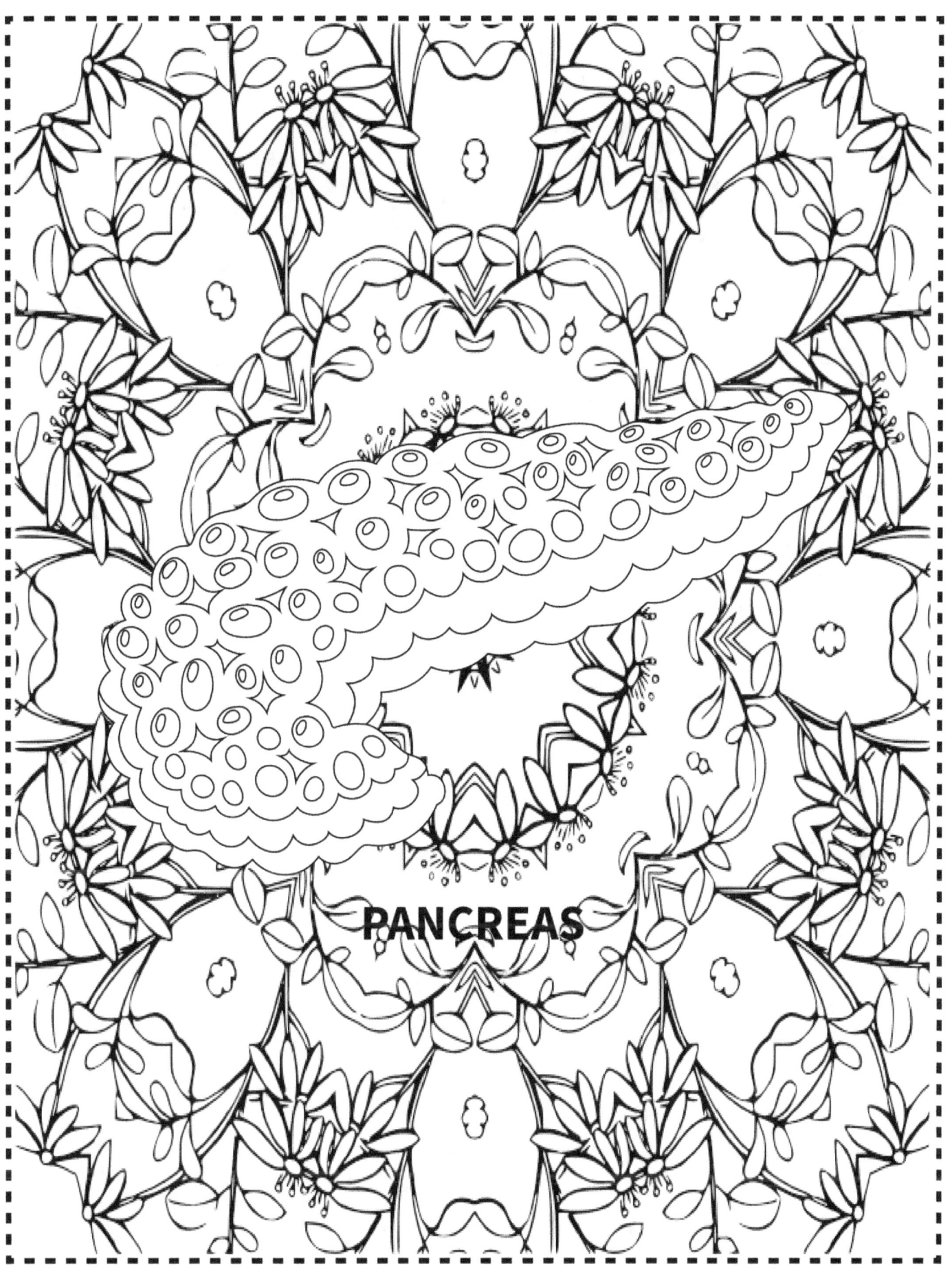

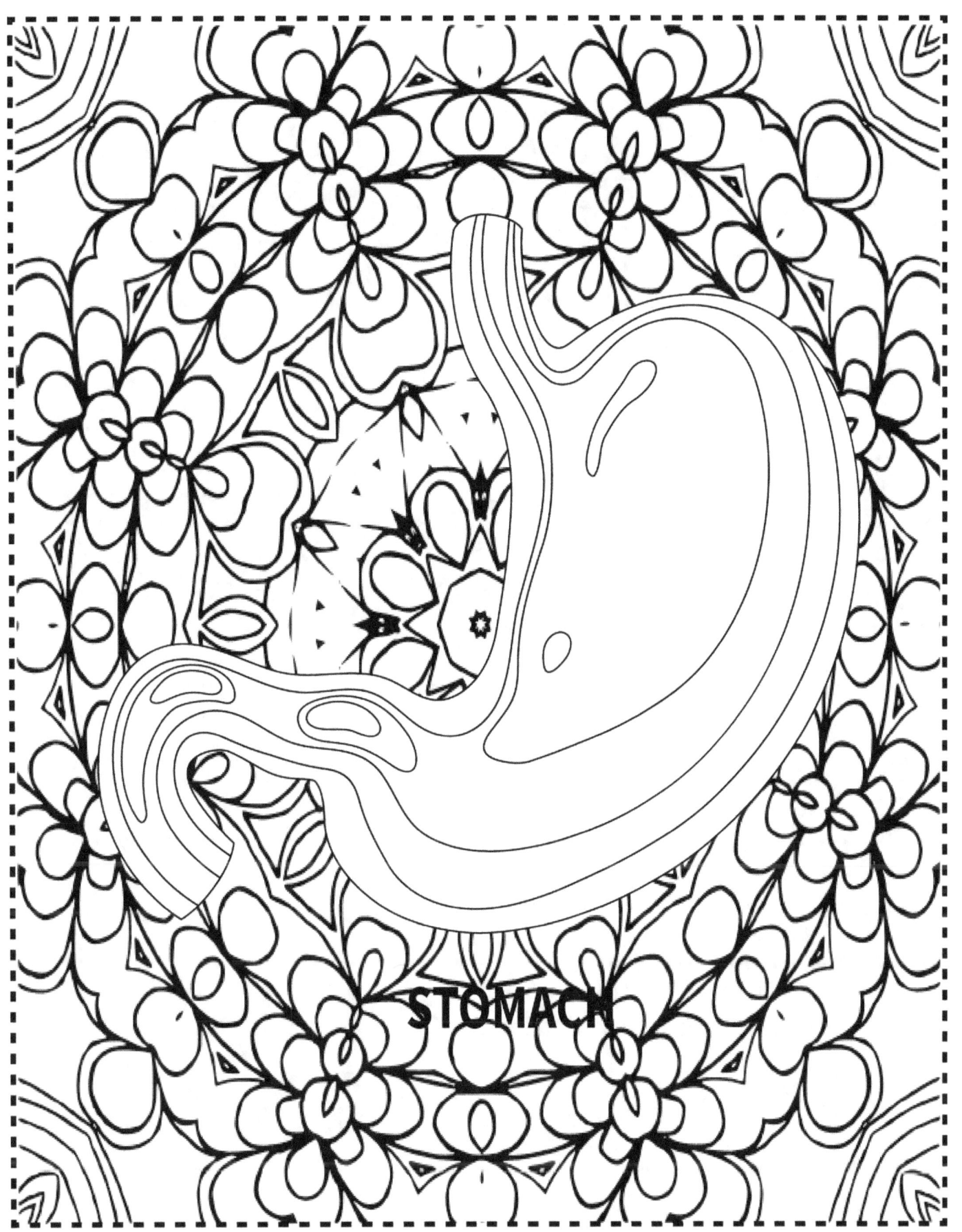

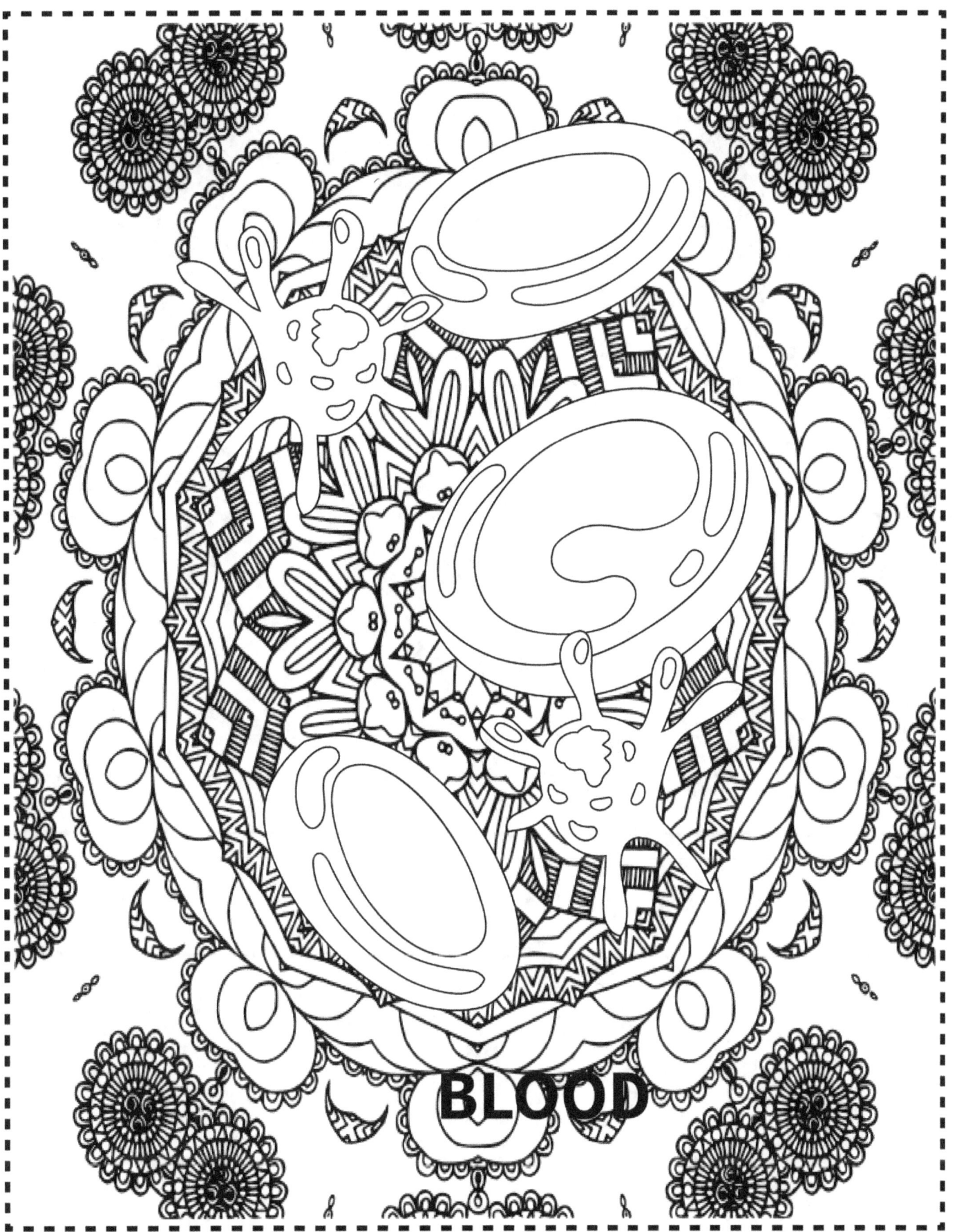

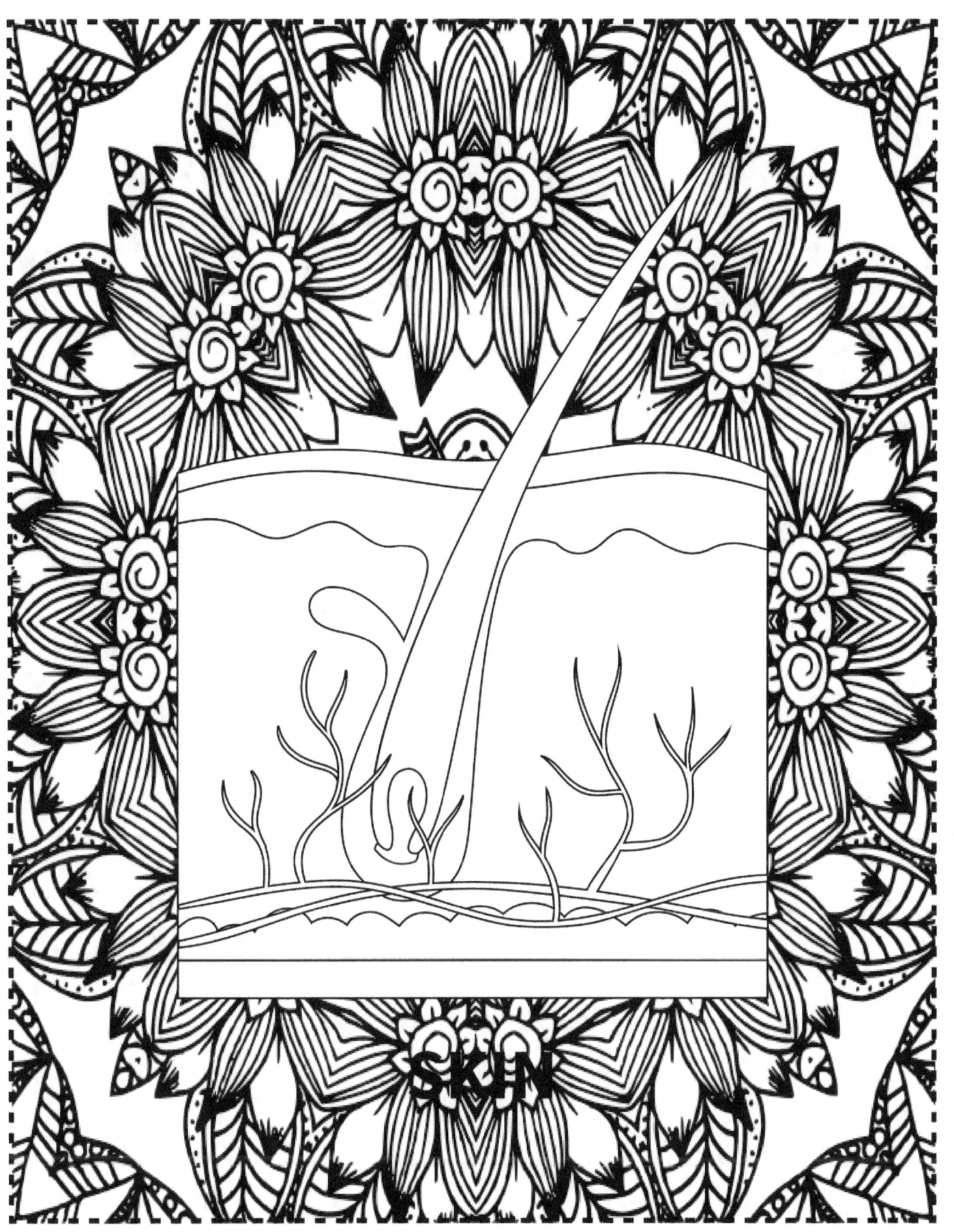

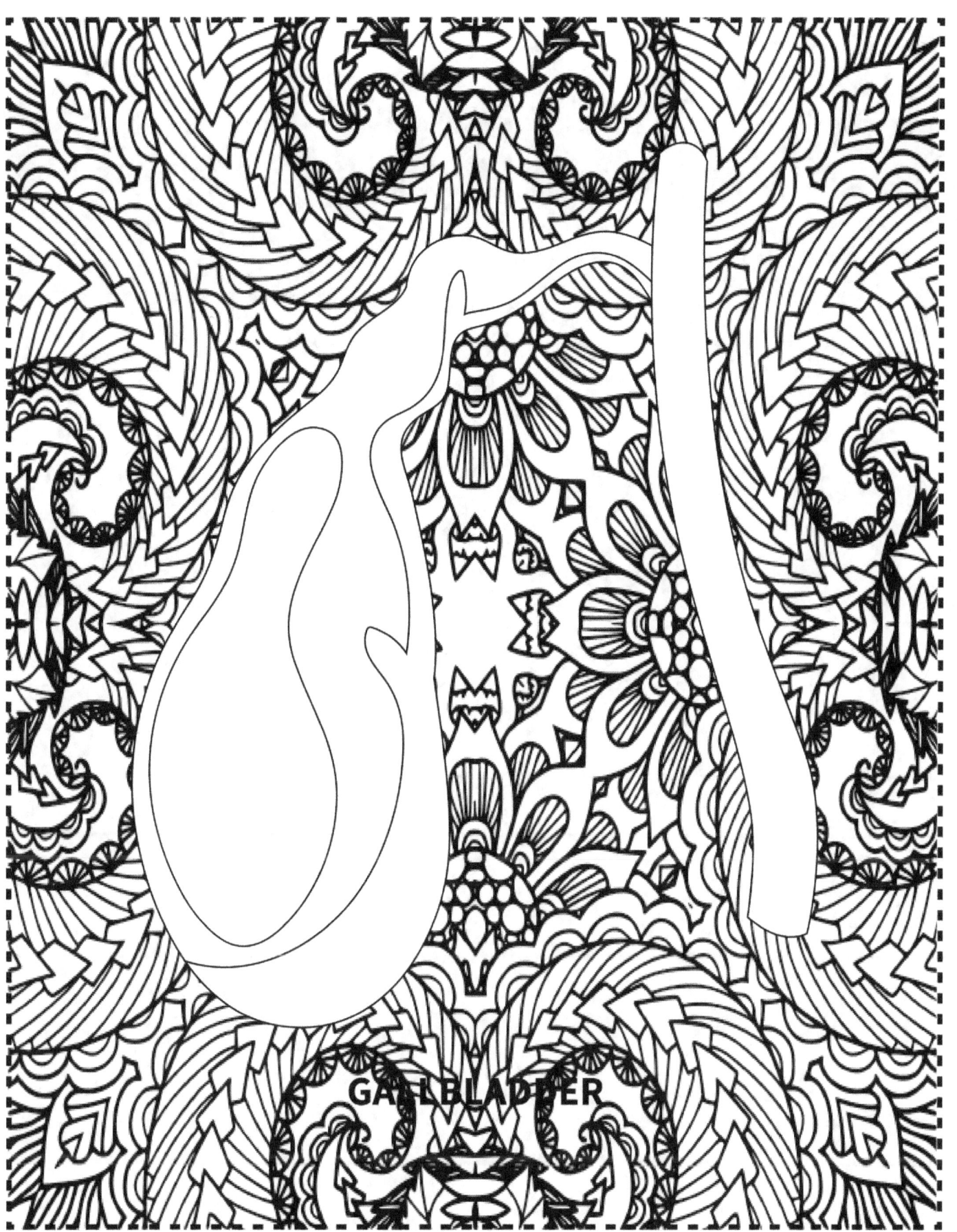

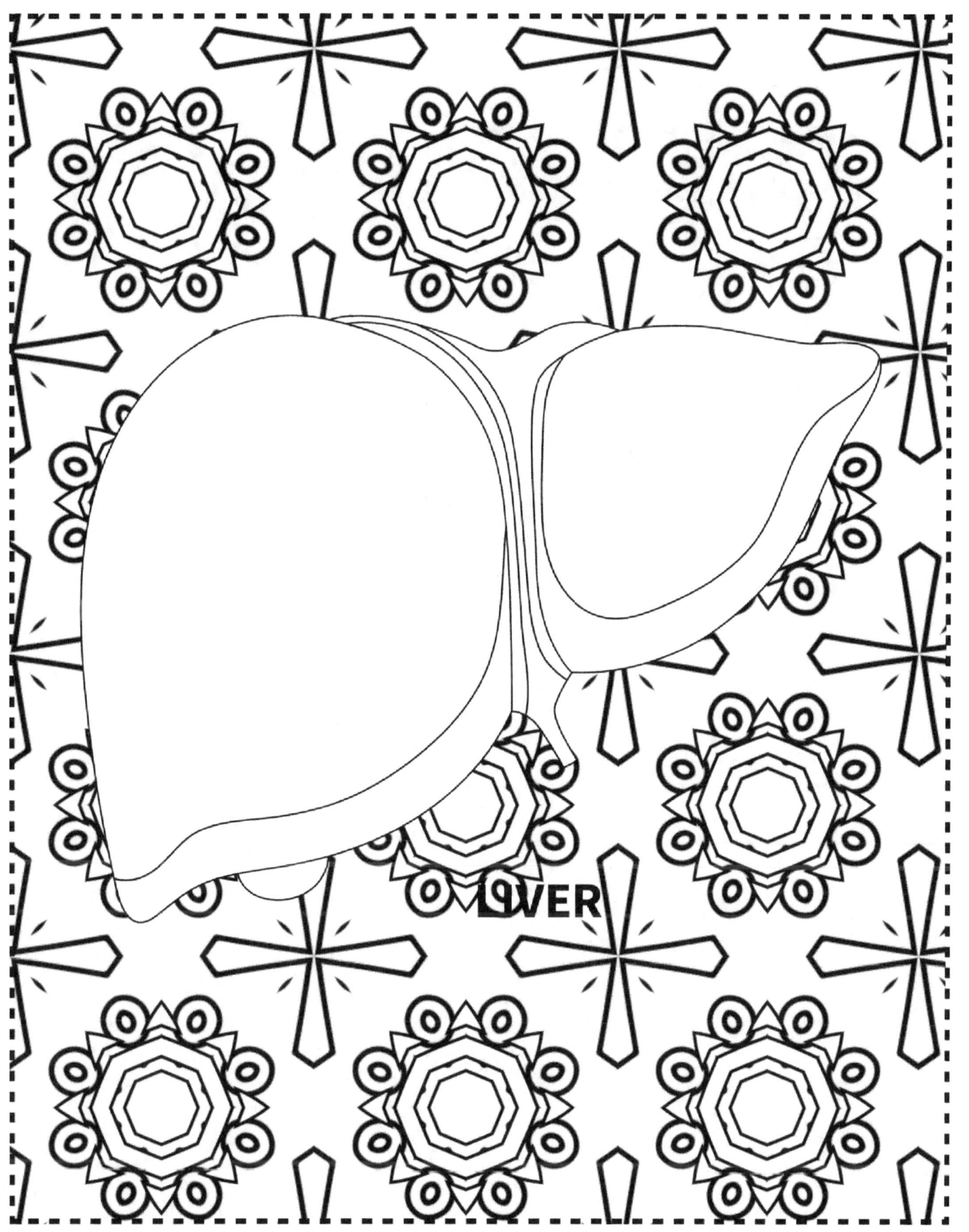

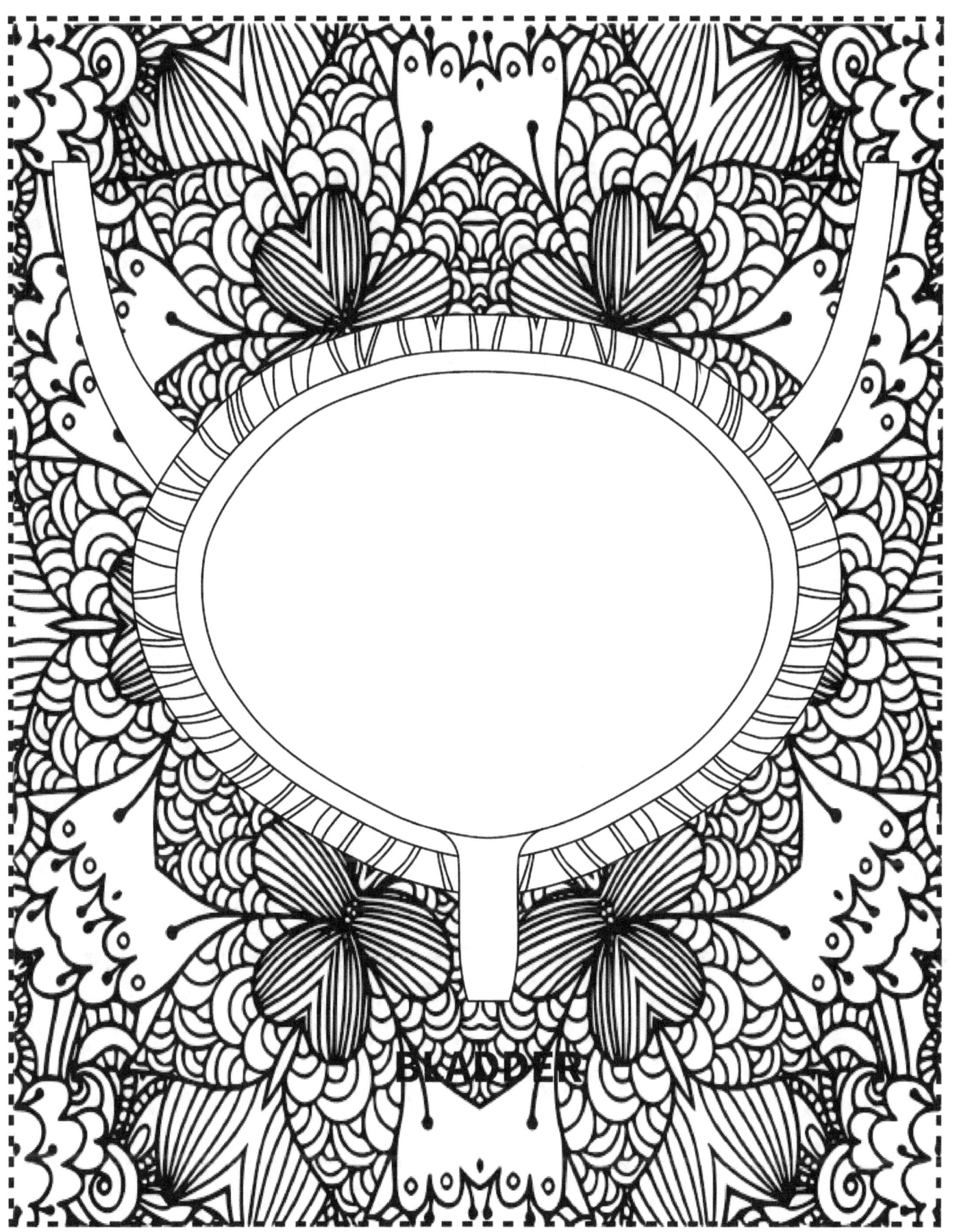

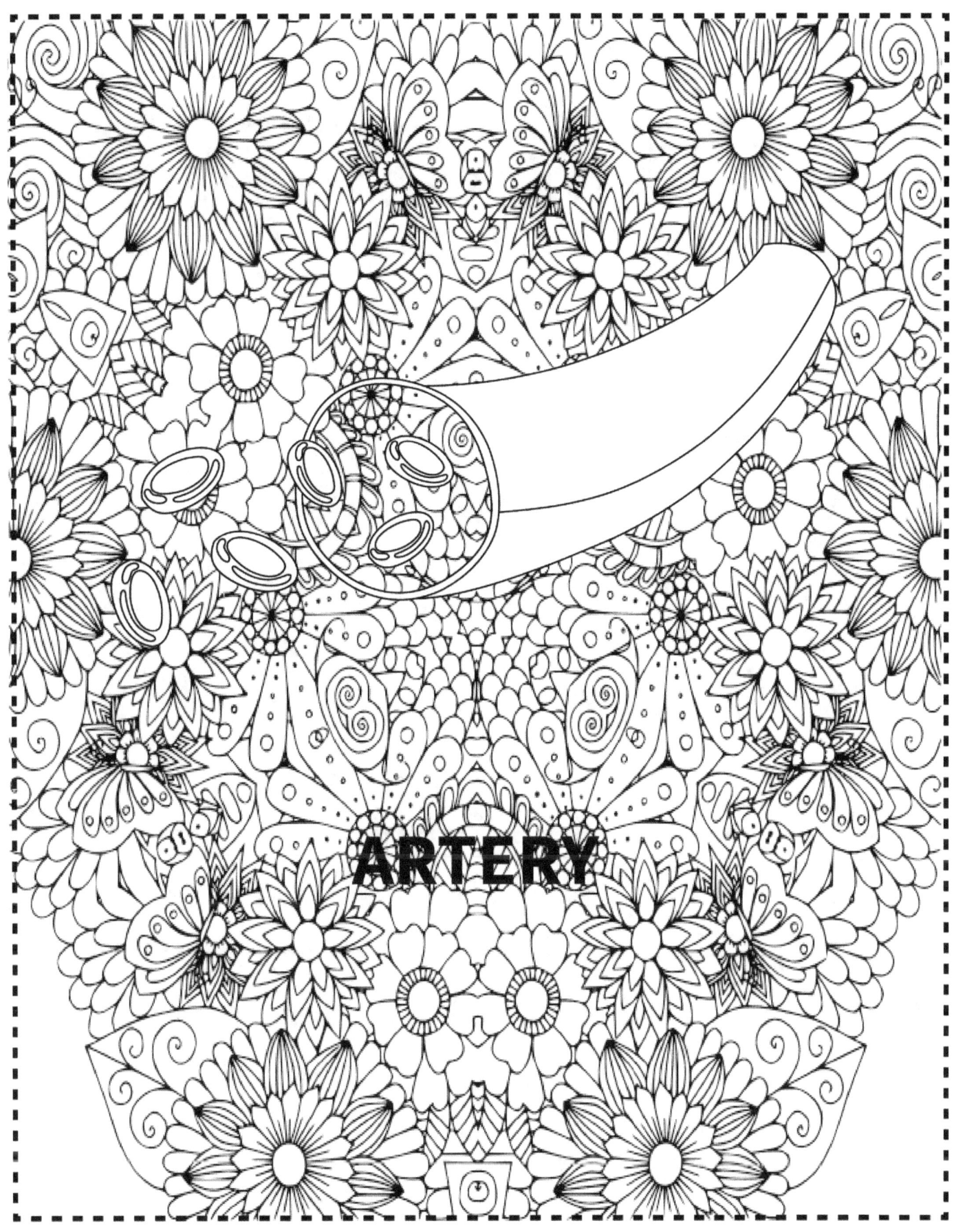

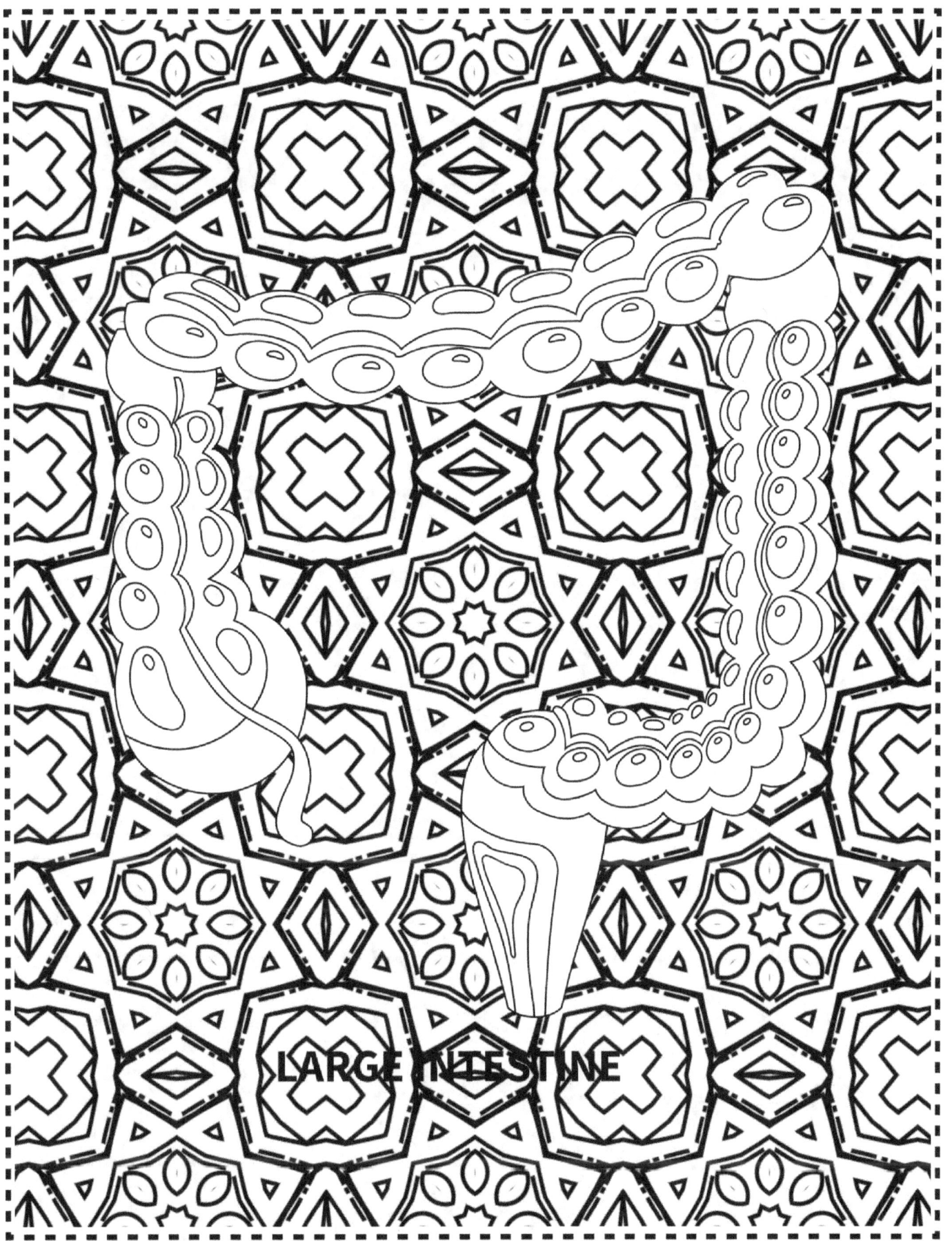

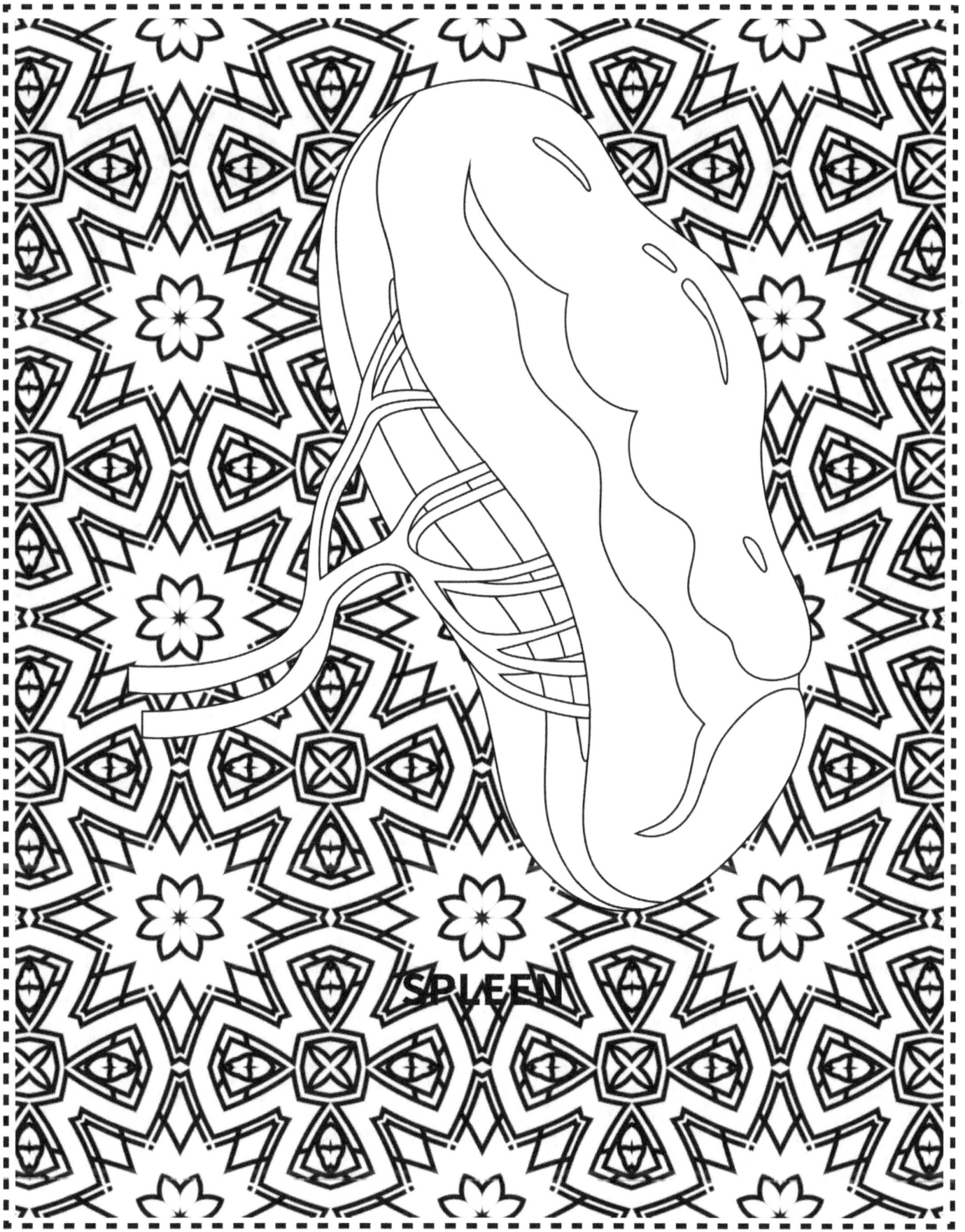

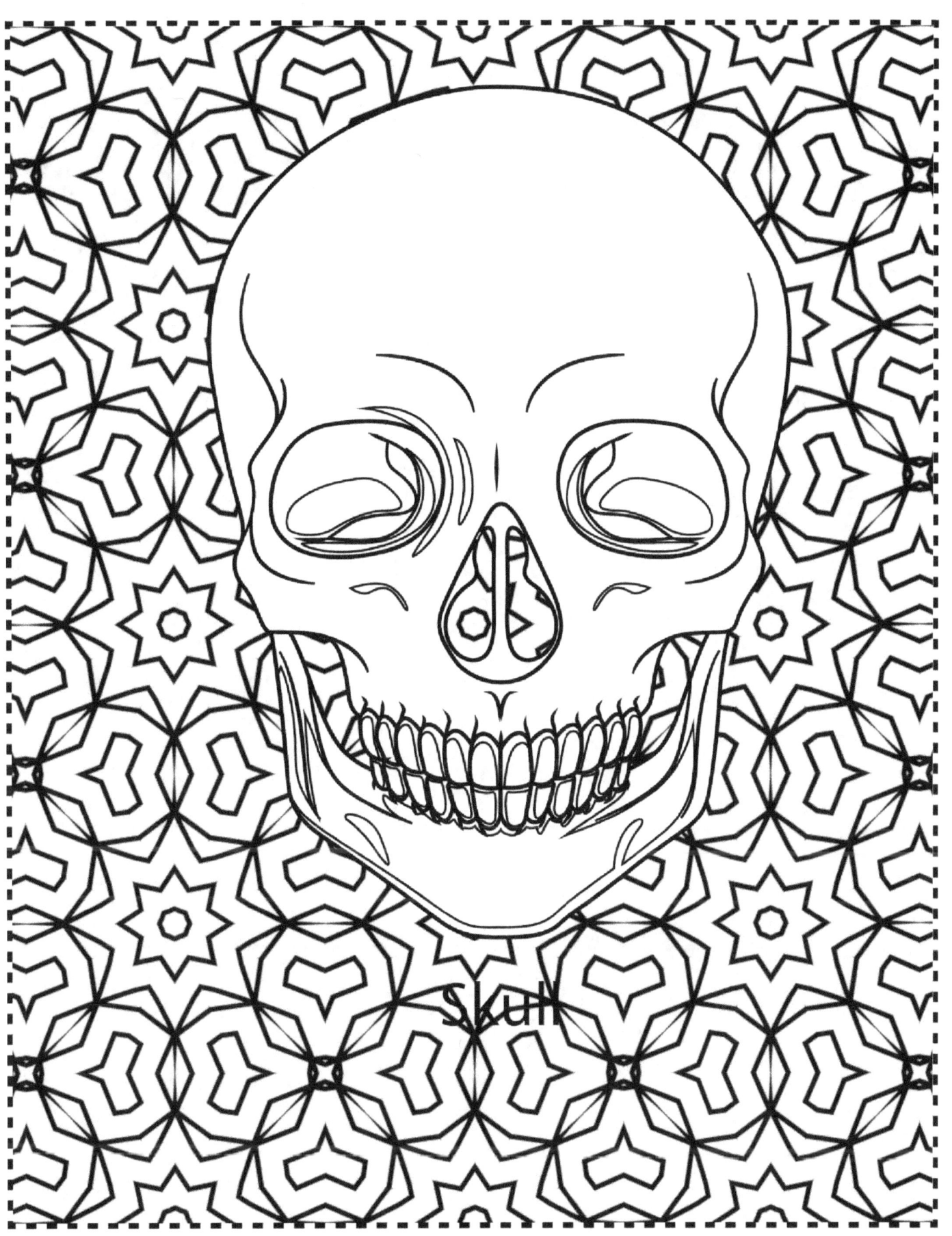

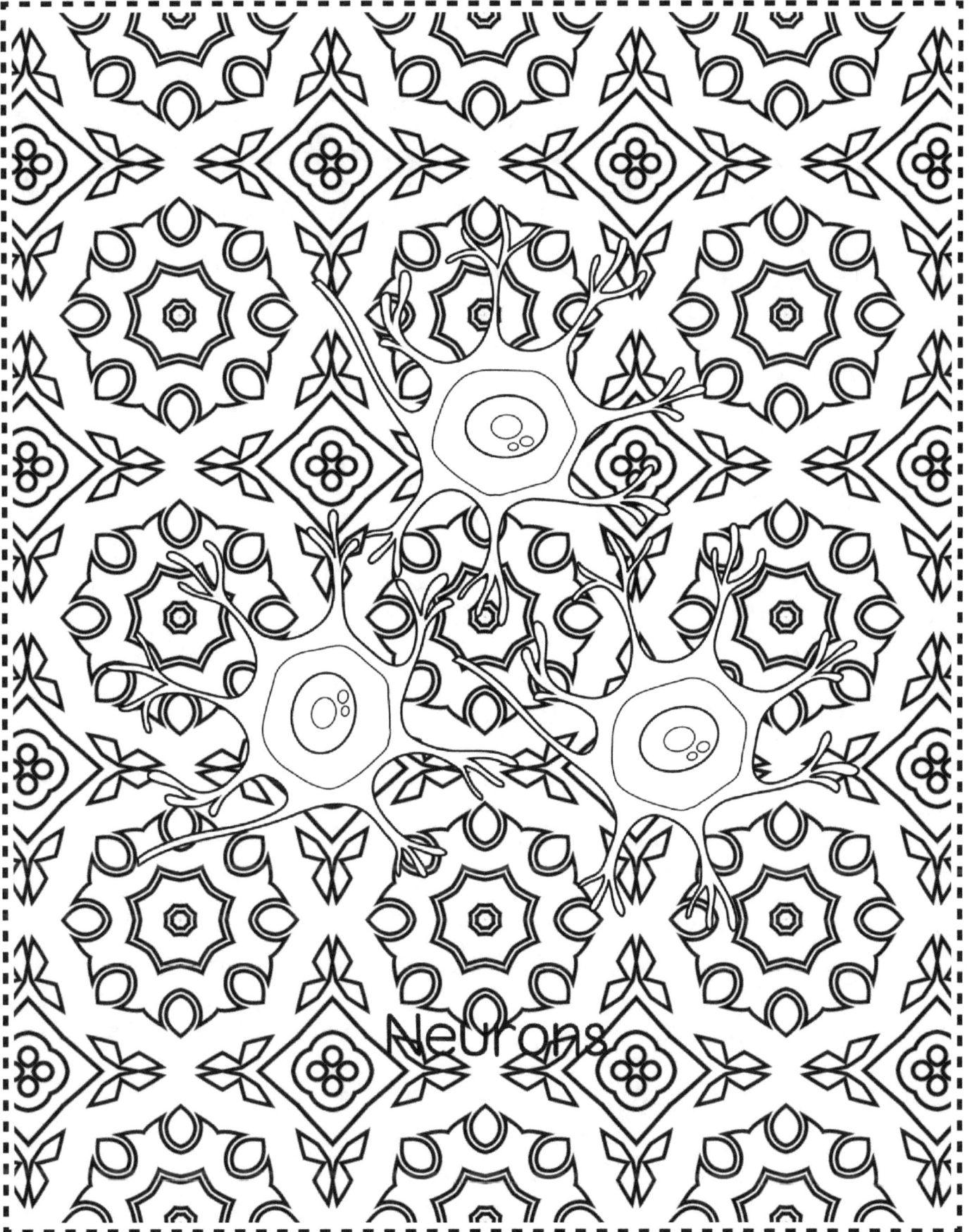

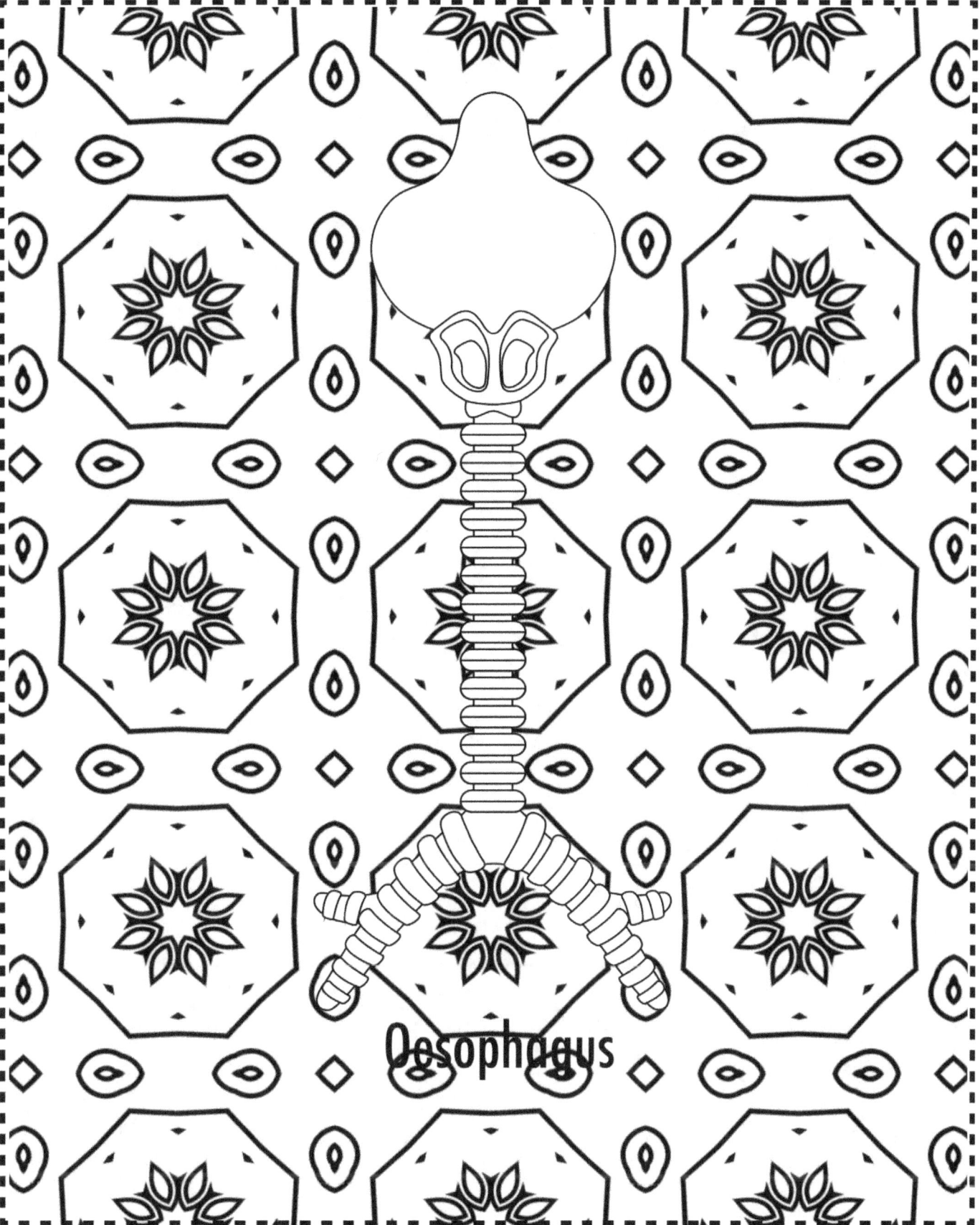

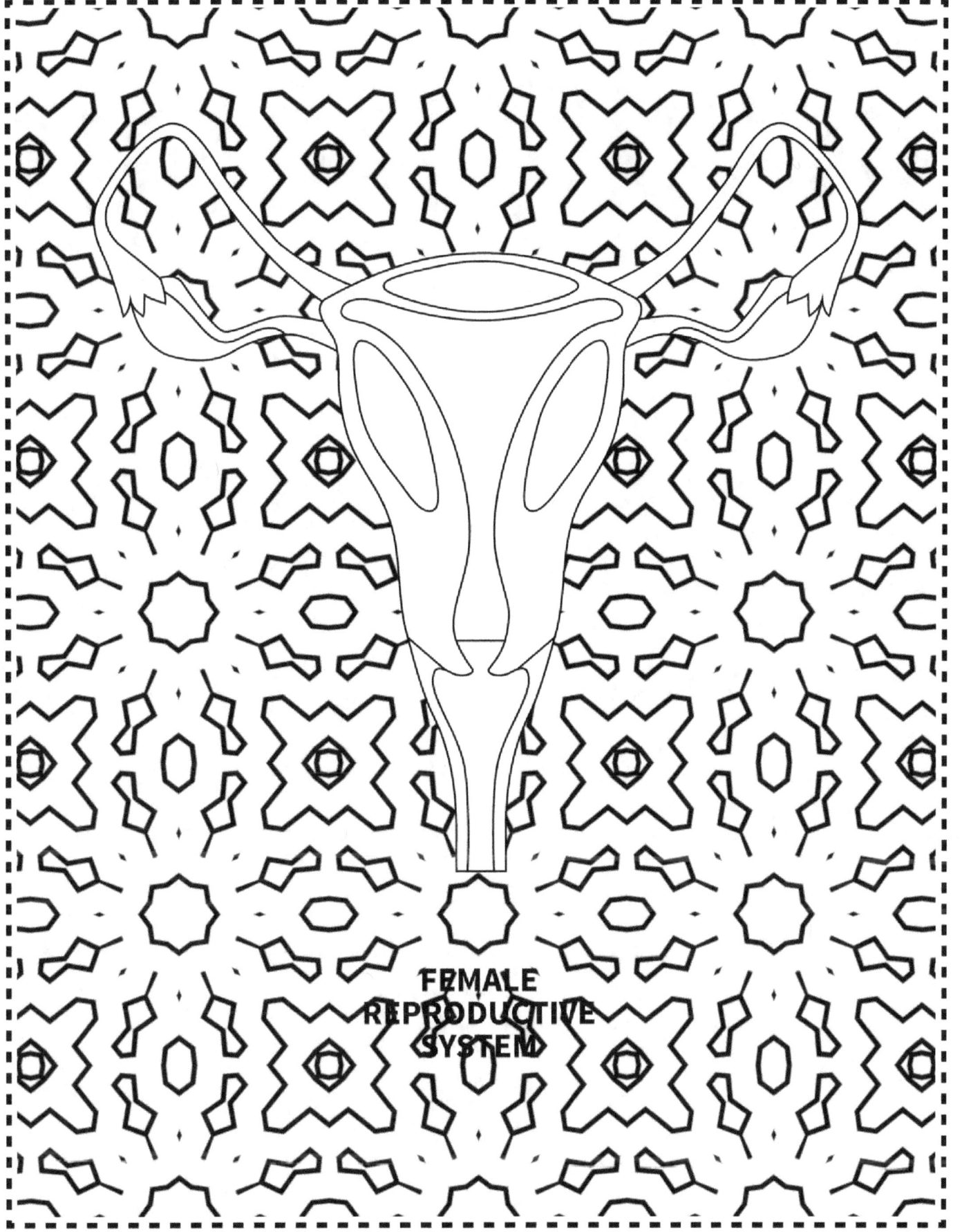

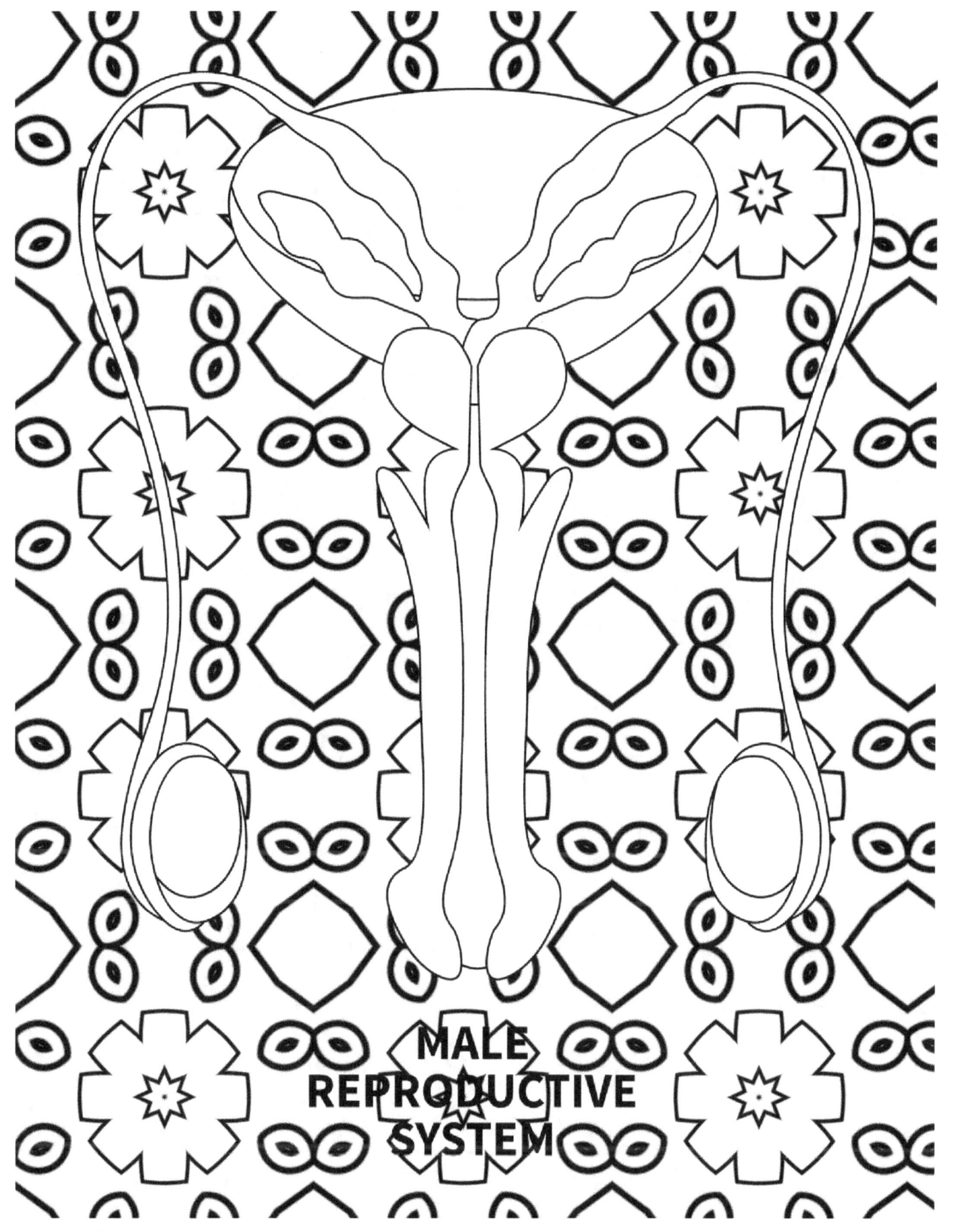

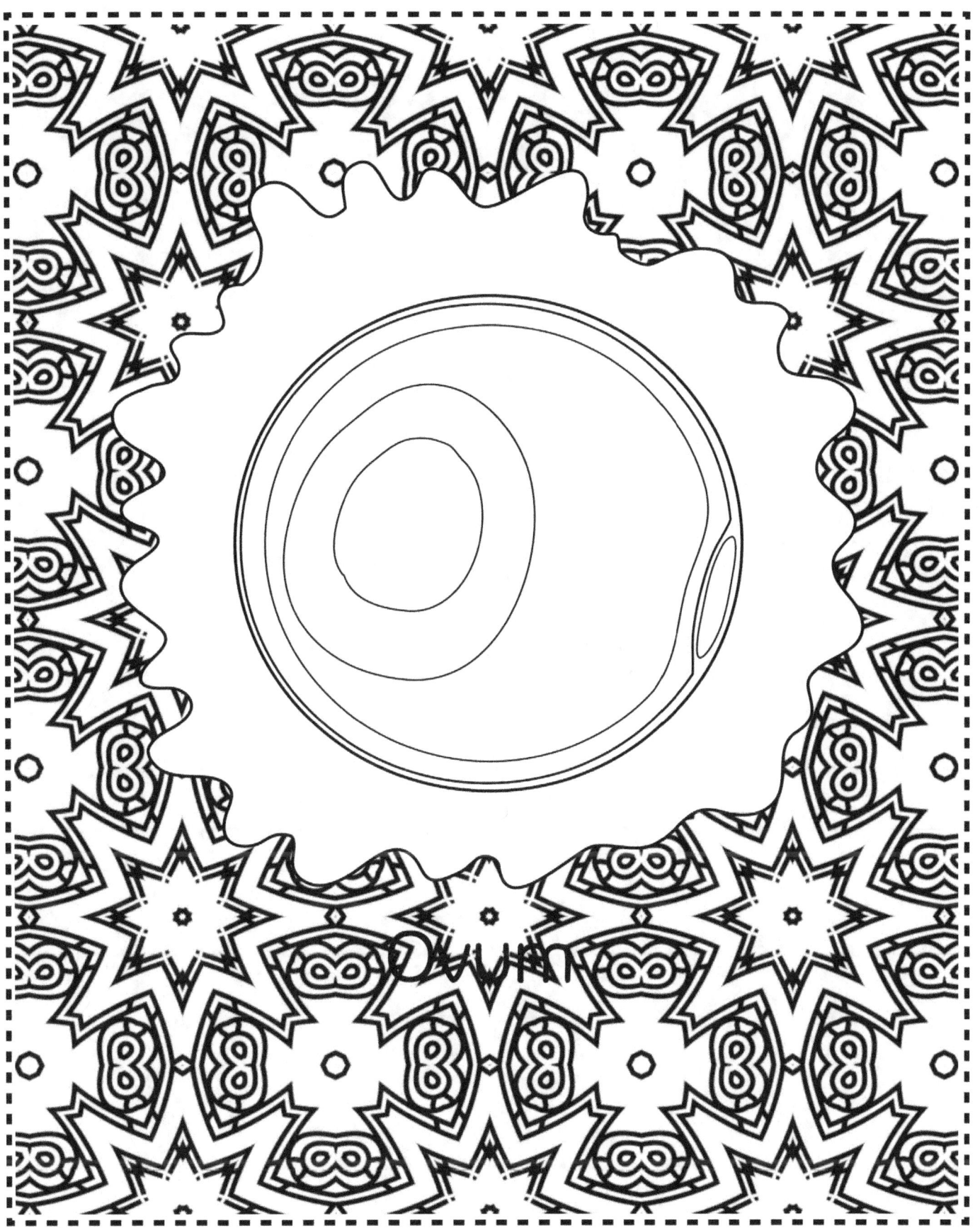

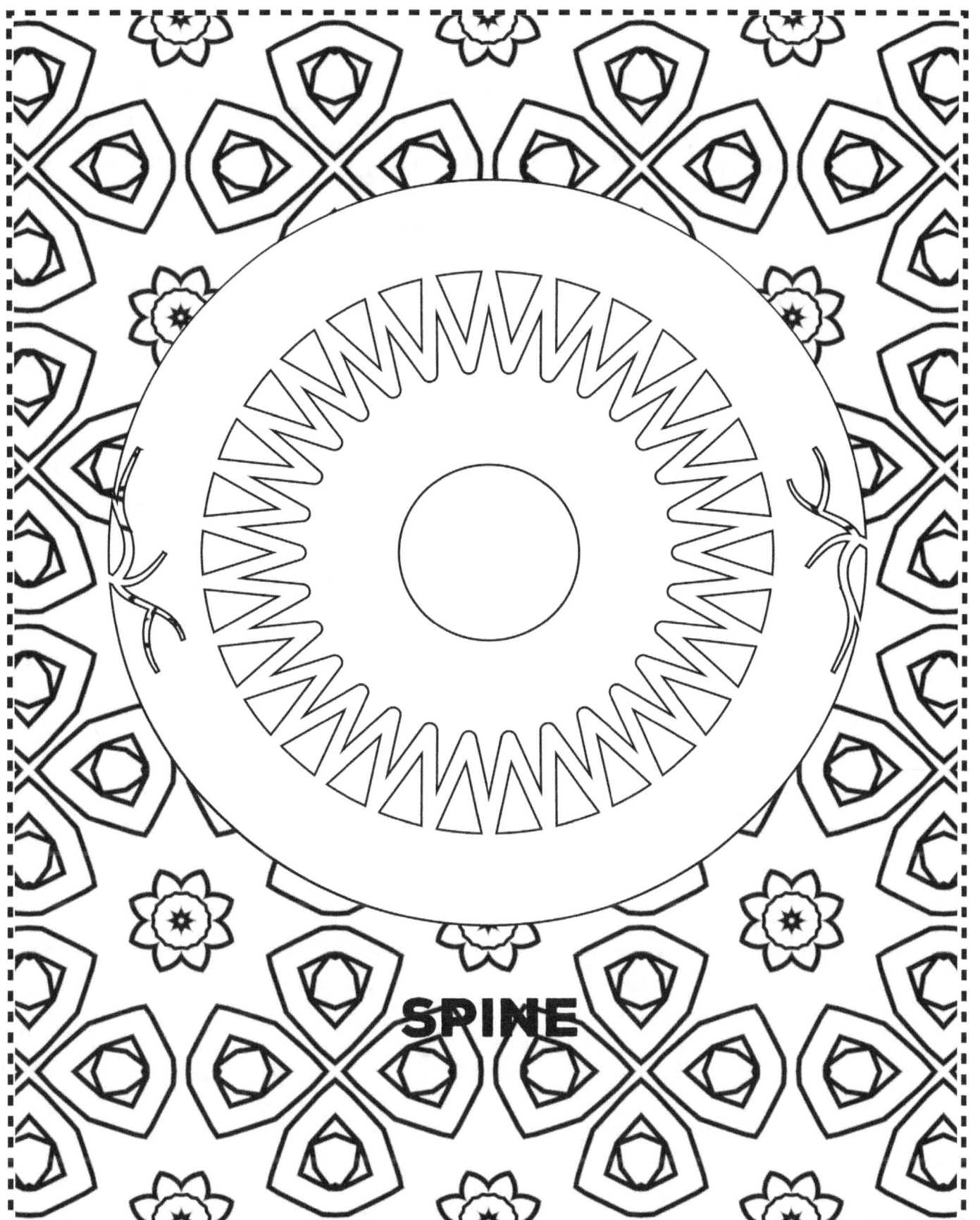

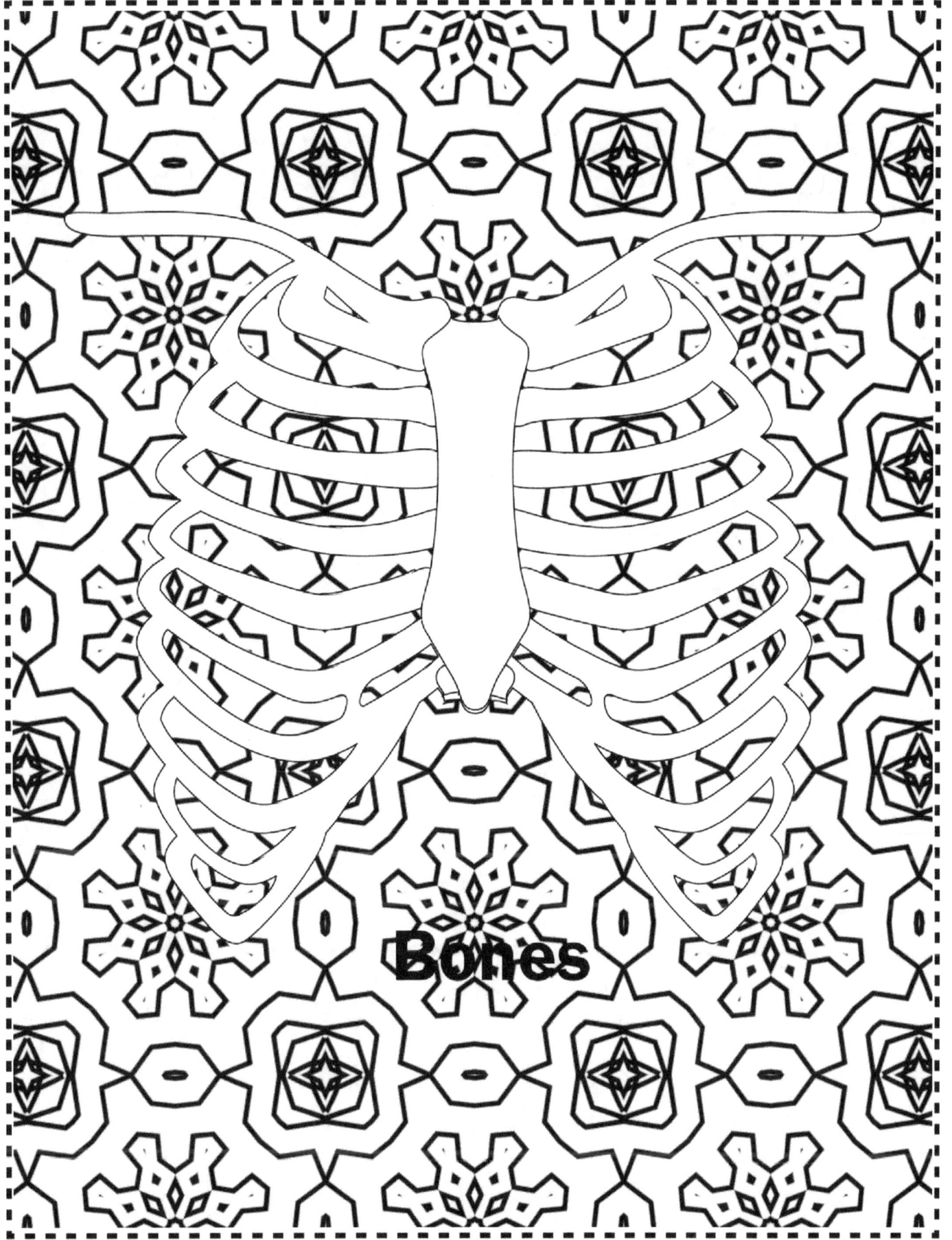

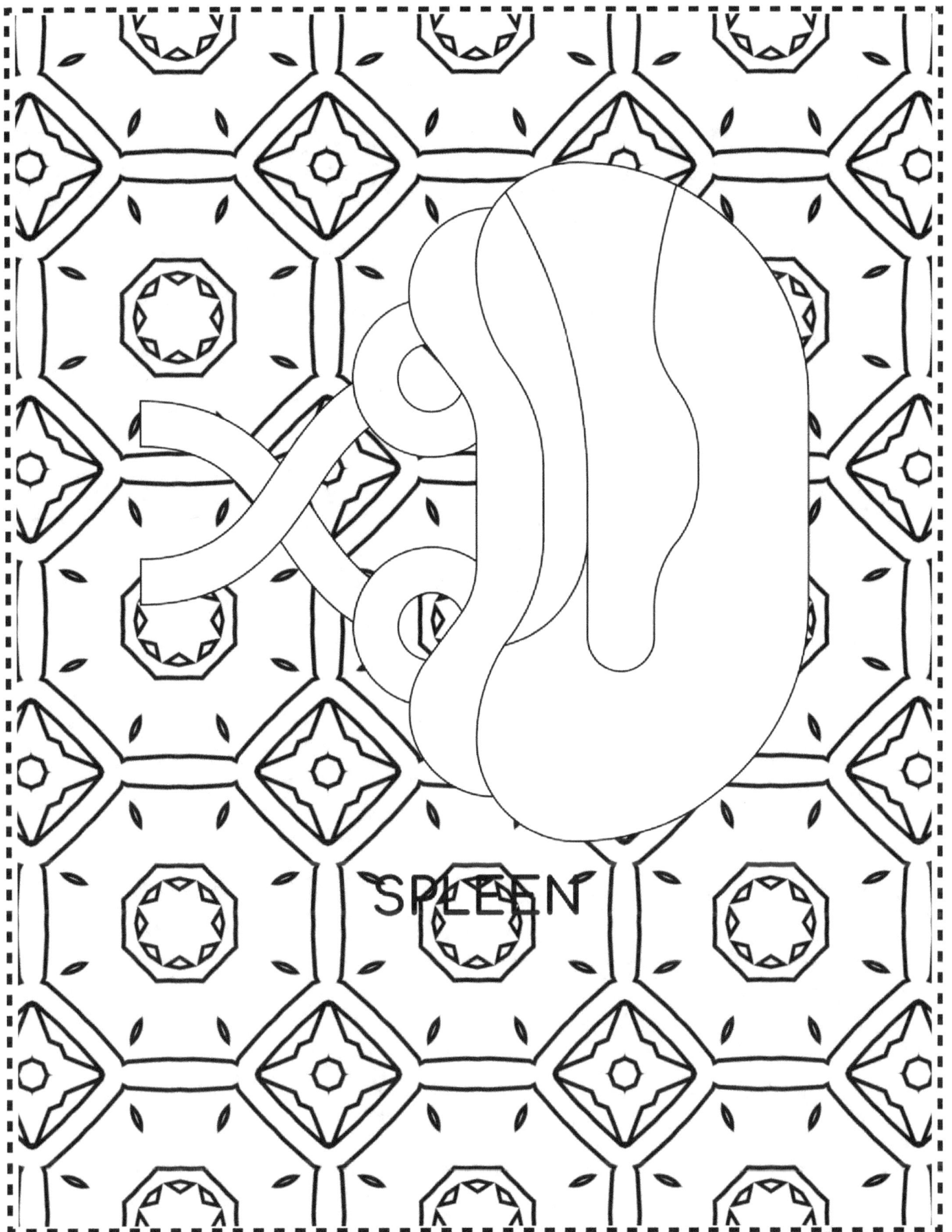

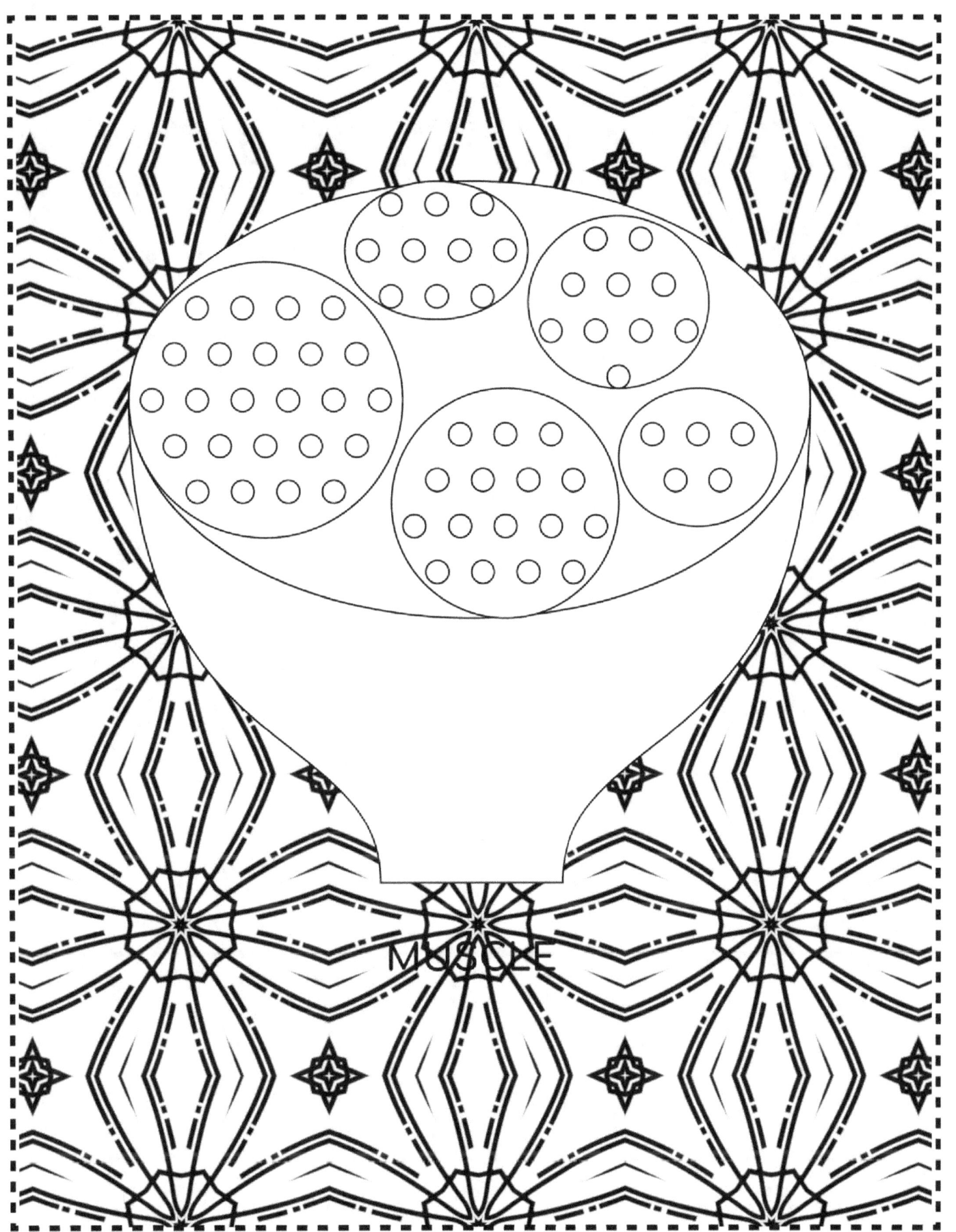

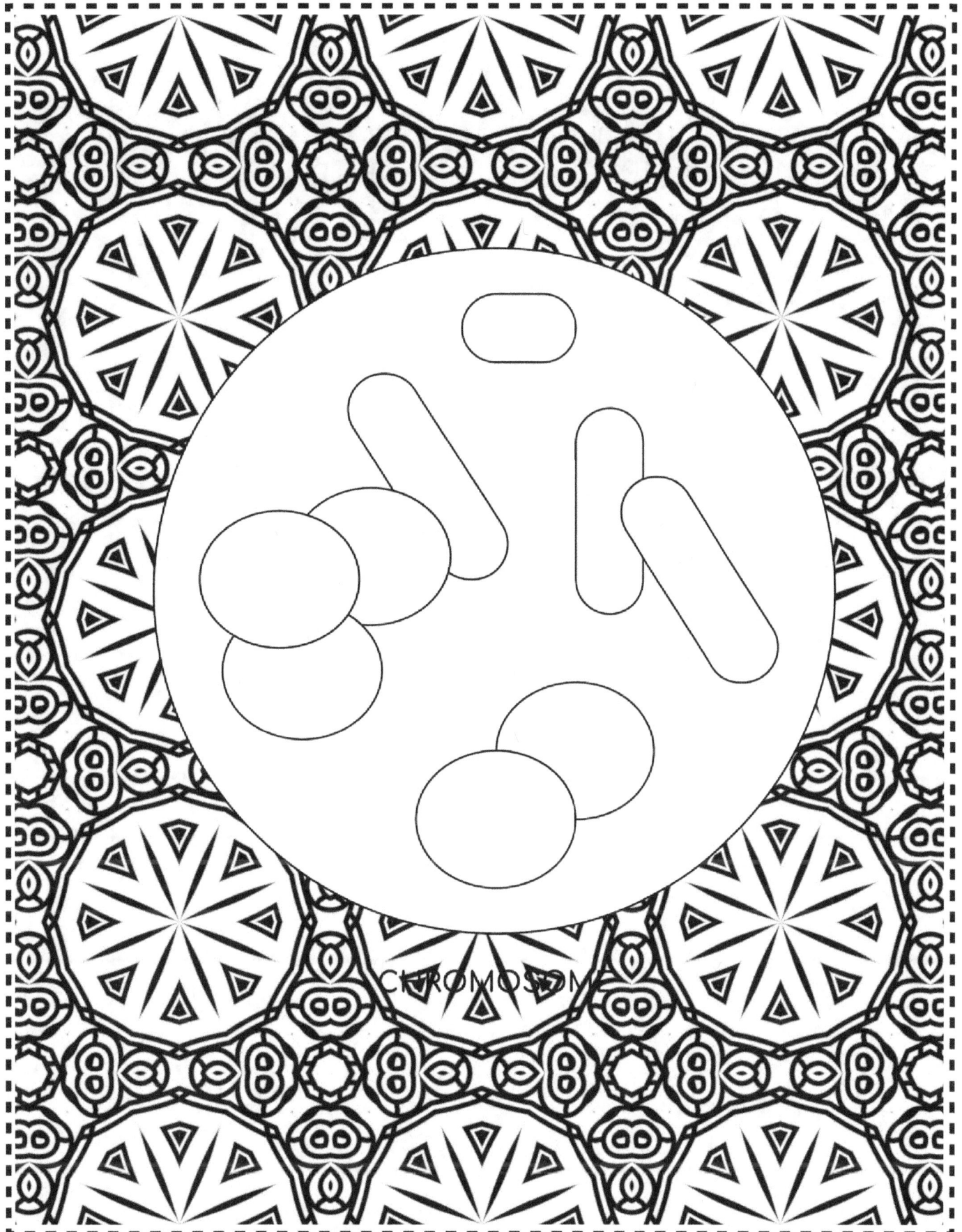

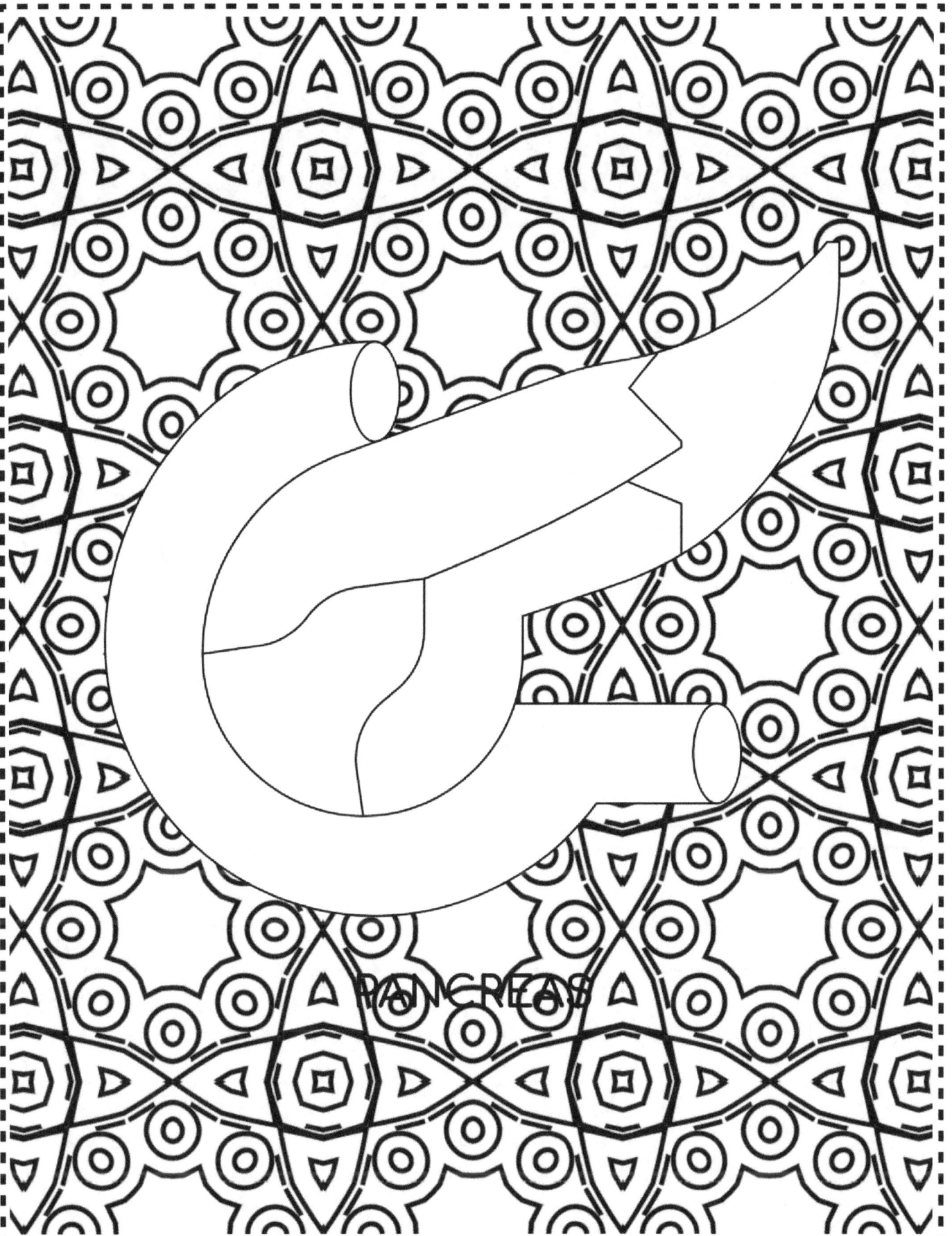

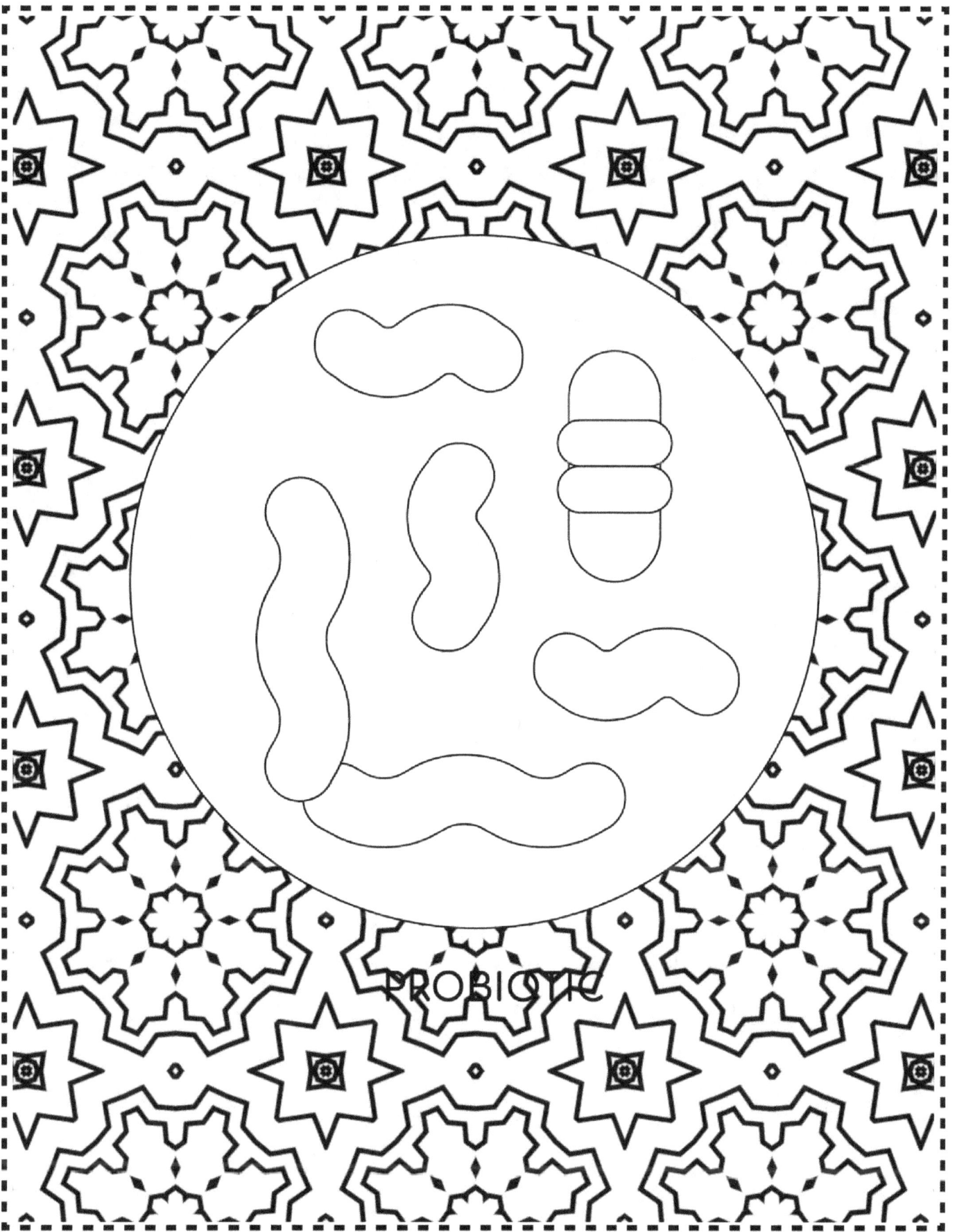
PROBIOTIC

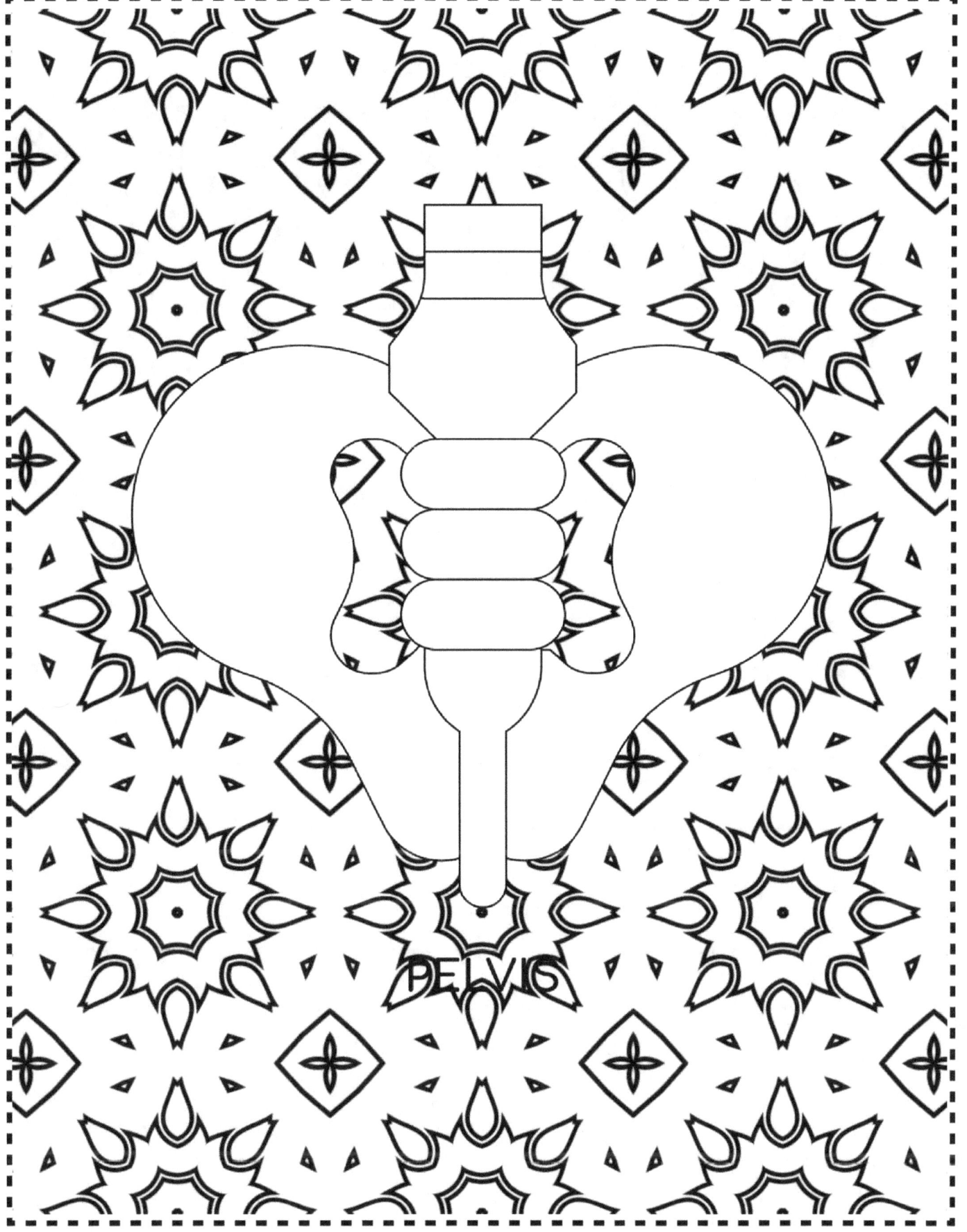

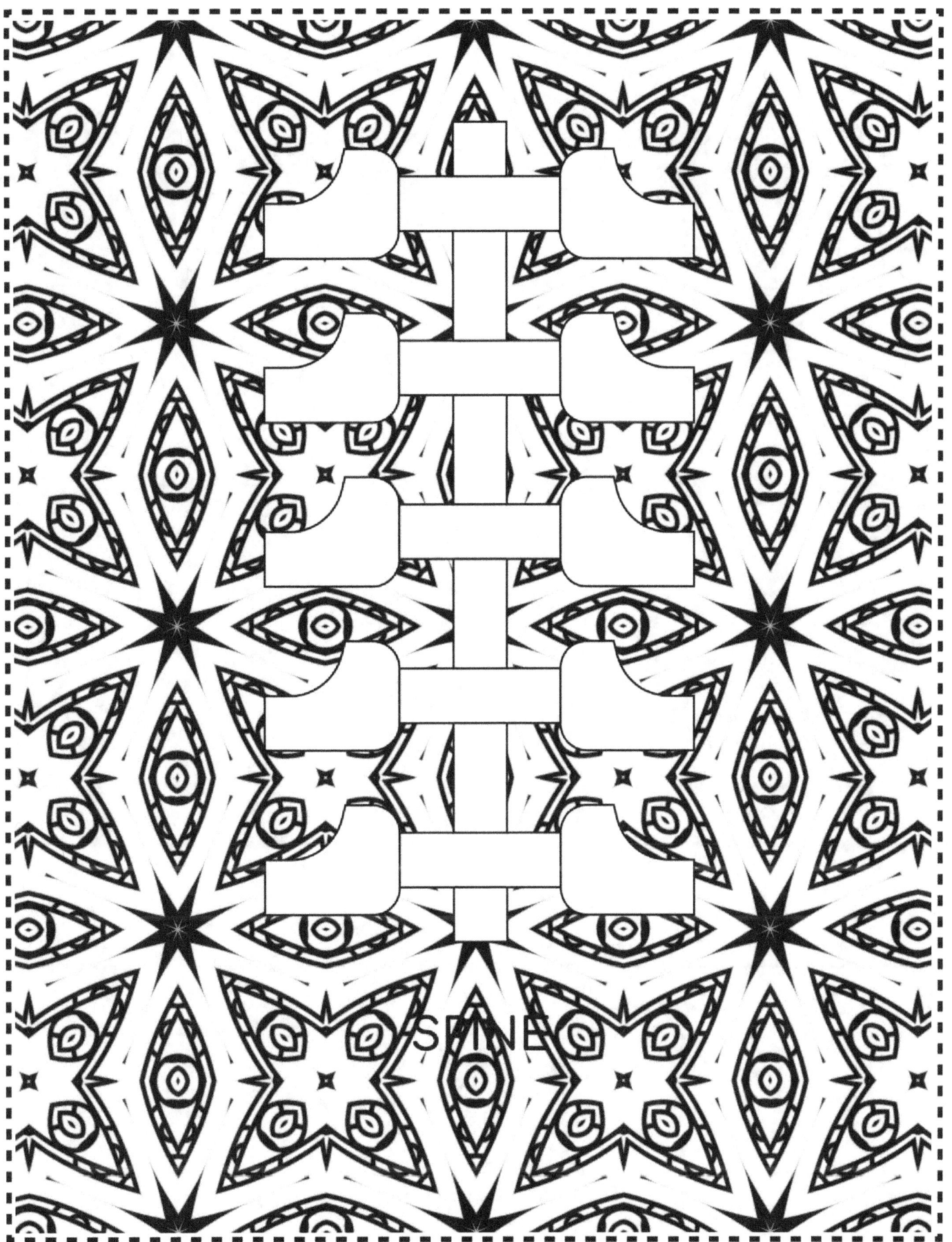

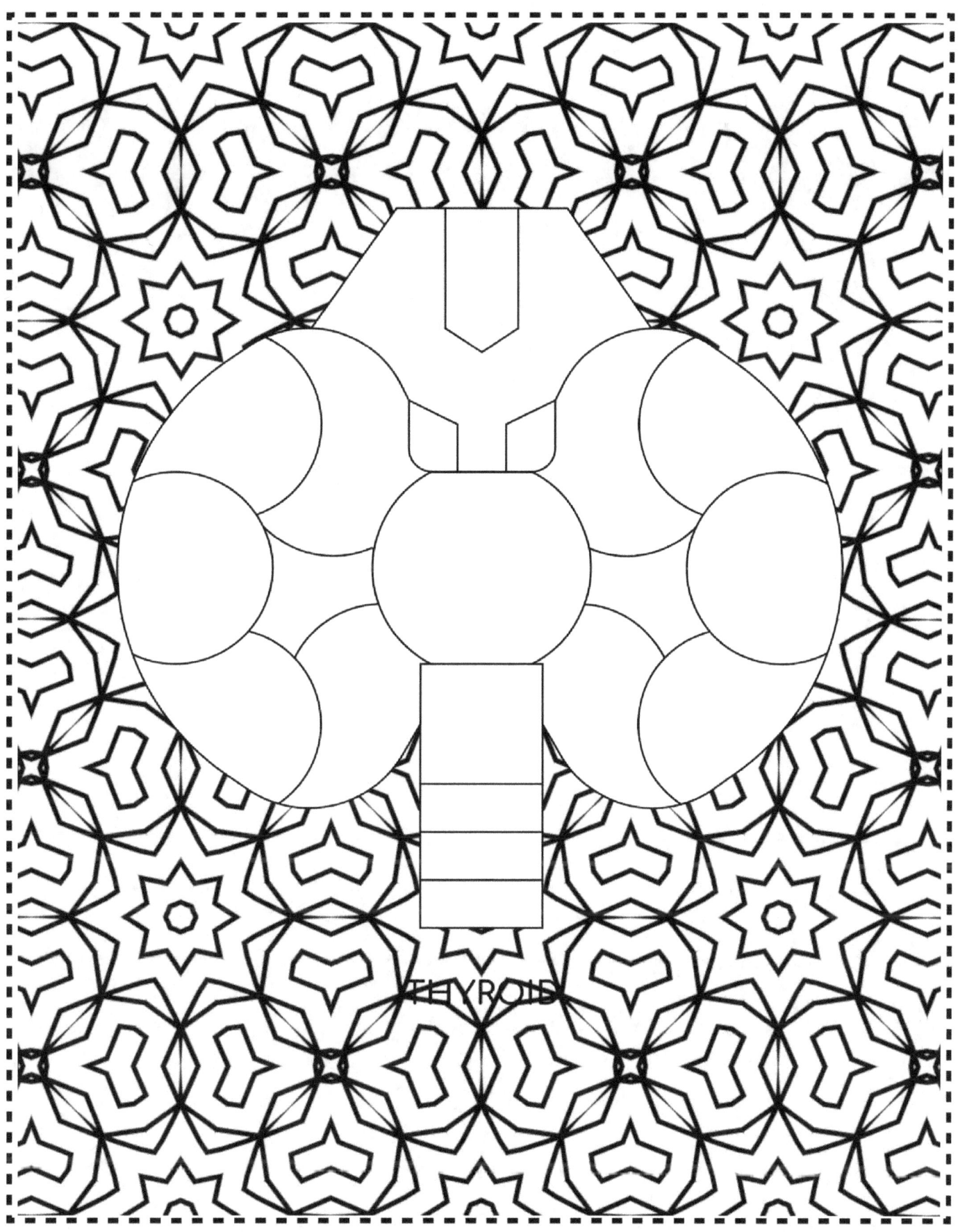

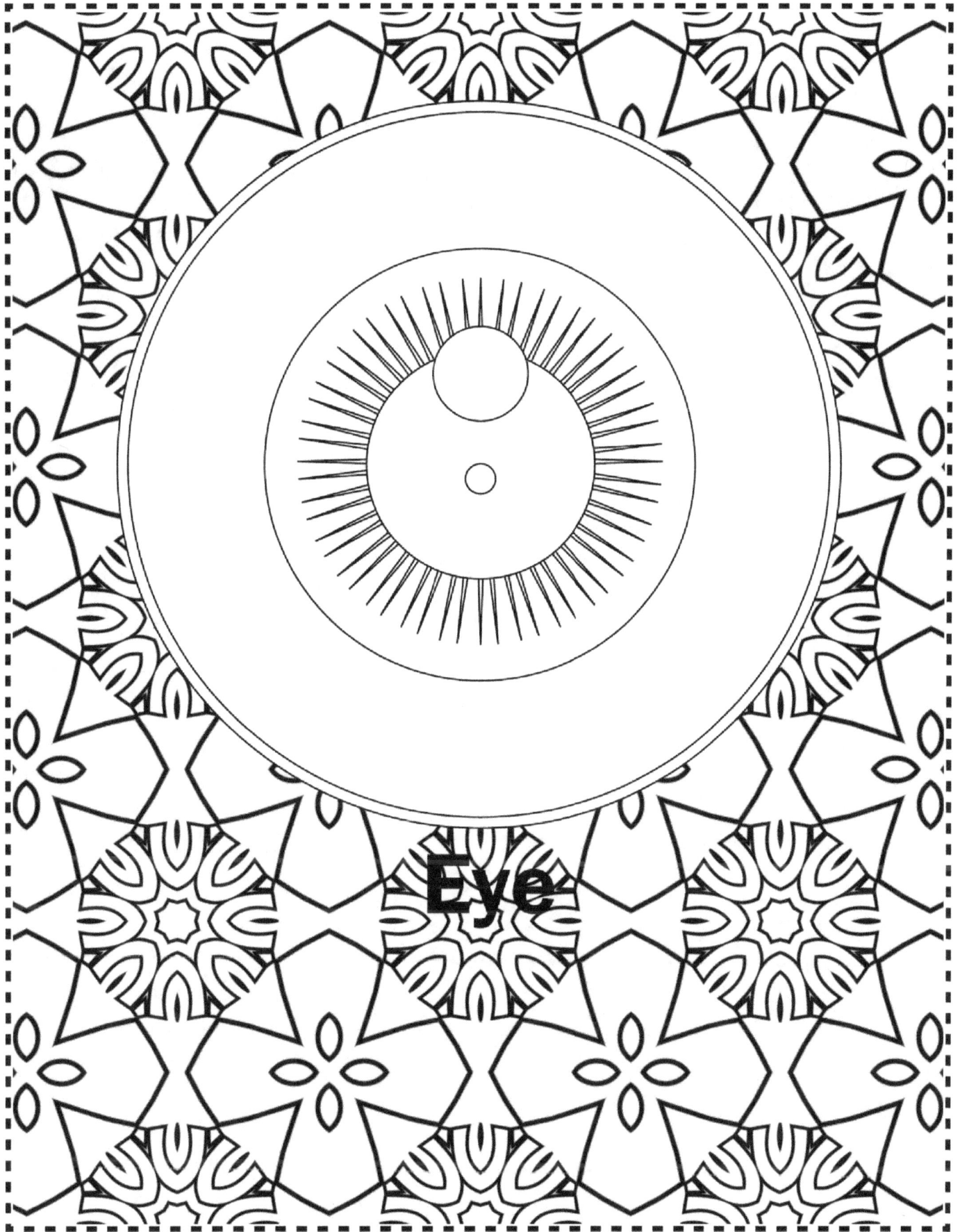

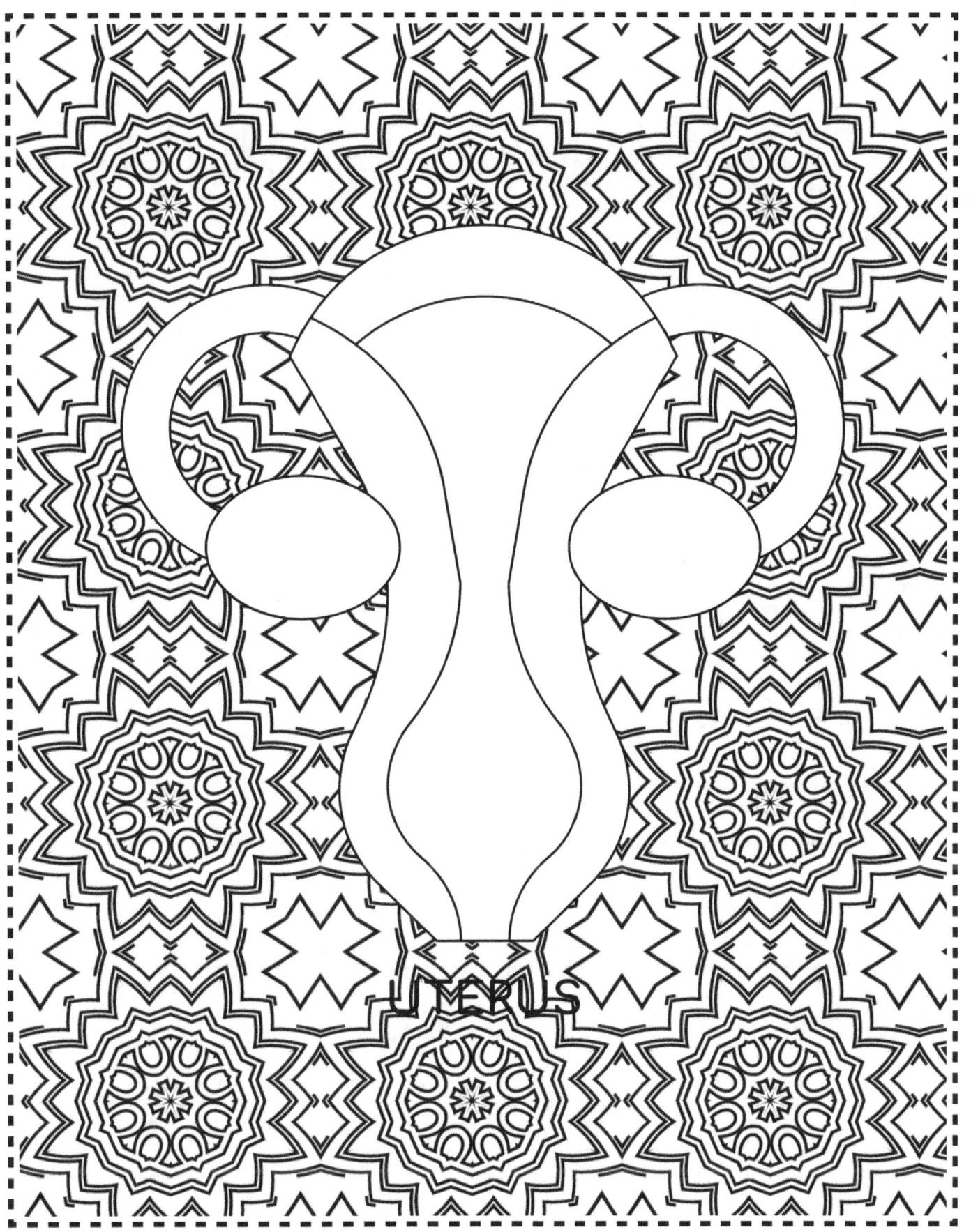

www.ingramcontent.com/pod-product-compliance
Lightning Source LLC
Chambersburg PA
CBHW080743240526
45472CB00025B/2216